Pre-hospital
Emergency
Medicine
at a Glance

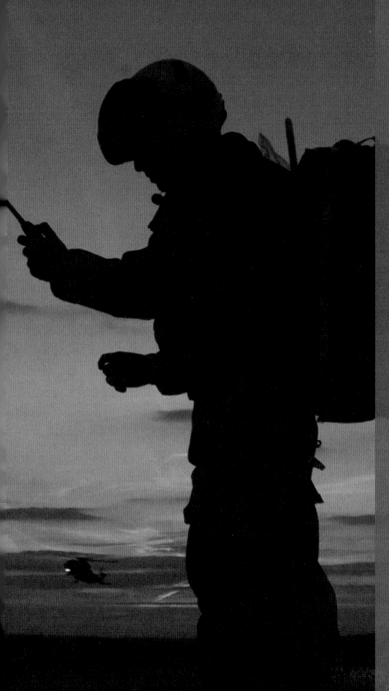

Pre-hospital Emergency Medicine at a Glance

Dr William Seligman
Core Anaesthetic Trainee
Imperial School of Anaesthesia

Dr Sameer Ganatra
Senior Resident Medical Officer
Intensive Care Medicine
Northern Sydney Local Health District

Dr Timothy Parker
Emergency Medicine Trainee
Australian College of Emergency Medicine
Northern New South Wales Local Health District

Dr Syed Masud
Consultant in Emergency Medicine & Pre-hospital
Emergency Medicine
Oxford University Hospitals NHS
Foundation Trust;
Clinical Governance Lead
Thames Valley Air Ambulance;
Senior Lecturer in Trauma and Pre-hospital
Emergency Medicine
University of Oxford

WILEY Blackwell

Registered Offices: John Wiley & Sons, Inc., 111 River Street, Hoboken, NJ 07030, USA
John Wiley & Sons, Ltd., The Atrium, Southern Gate, Chichester, West Sussex, PO19 8SQ, UK

Editorial Office: 9600 Garsington Road, Oxford, OX4 2DQ, UK

For details of our global editorial offices, customer services and more information about Wiley products, visit us at www.wiley.com.

Wiley also publishes its books in a variety of electronic formats and by print-on-demand. Some content that appears in standard print versions of this book may not be available in other formats.

Limit of Liability/Disclaimer of Warranty

Library of Congress Cataloging-in-Publication Data

Names: Seligman, William, 1990- author. | Ganatra, Sameer, author. | Parker, Timothy, 1989- author. | Masud, Syed, 1972- author.
Title: Pre-hospital emergency medicine at a glance / William Seligman, Sameer Ganatra, Timothy Parker, Syed Masud.
Other titles: At a glance series (Oxford, England).
Description: Hoboken, NJ : John Wiley & Sons Ltd, 2018. | Series: At a glance series | Includes index.
Identifiers: LCCN 2017000447 (print) | LCCN 2017001693 (ebook) | ISBN 9781118829929 (pbk.) | ISBN 9781118829950 (Adobe PDF) | ISBN 9781118829967 (ePub)
Subjects: | MESH: Emergency Medical Services—methods | Emergency Treatment—methods | Emergencies | Critical Care—methods | Handbooks
Classification: LCC RC86.8 (print) | LCC RC86.8 (ebook) | NLM WB 39 | DDC 616.02/5—dc23
LC record available at https://lccn.loc.gov/2017000447

Cover image: Courtesy of Syed Masud

Set in 9.5/11.5 Minion Pro by Aptara Inc., New Delhi, India
Printed and bound in Singapore by Markono Print Media Pte Ltd

10 9 8 7 6 5 4 3 2 1

Contents

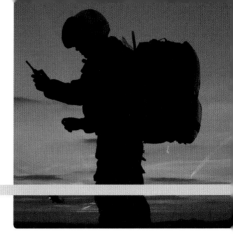

Preface

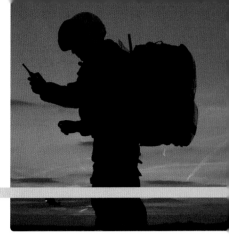

Pre-hospital Emergency Medicine is an innovative and exciting new sub-specialty that is saving lives and has great potential to change the way medicine is practised. The sub-specialty has grown exponentially since its inception and has enormous potential to answer research questions that will benefit patients both outside and within the hospital.

Although it has a short history, we must remember that the sub-specialty emerged not only from the ambulance service but also from doctors who decided to travel to patients on the roadside with limited equipment, in order to deliver whatever care they could. It is from these humble beginnings that the sub-specialty has developed into the incredibly influential model of care seen today in modern pre-hospital emergency units.

With great admiration and respect, I would like to thank those that developed the concepts that made Pre-hospital Emergency Medicine the force for good that is today.

We must never forget that the practice of Pre-hospital Emergency Medicine is a sacrifice not only for those who deliver care but also for their loved ones who, in turn, care for them. Without family and friends, we would be unable to deliver the quality of care that is expected in the challenging pre-hospital environment. We are too quick to forget the partners who wait in the middle of the night for their loved ones to return from road traffic accidents or other serious incidents to deliver comforting words and understanding. Without them, we couldn't do what we do.

This book is dedicated to both those who deliver what I like to believe is the 'bungee jumping' of medicine, and to those who silently support them in the background.

Dr Syed Masud
Consultant in Emergency Medicine & Pre-hospital
Emergency Medicine, Oxford University Hospitals NHS
Foundation Trust;
Clinical Governance Lead, Thames Valley Air Ambulance;
Senior Lecturer in Trauma and Pre-Hospital Emergency
Medicine, University of Oxford

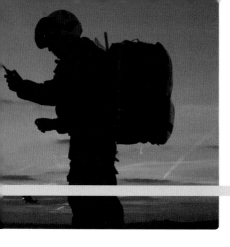

Contributors

Chapter 14: The difficult airway
Dr Adam Fendius
Consultant in Trauma Anaesthesia
Oxford University Hospitals NHS Foundation Trust

Dr Edward Horwell
Core Surgical Trainee
Wessex Deanery

Chapter 23: Paediatric trauma
Chapter 24: Trauma in the pregnant woman
Chapter 25: Trauma in the elderly
Dr Anna Barrow
Specialty Trainee in Anaesthesia and Intensive Care;
National Grid Trainee in Paediatric Intensive Care
Oxford Deanery

Chapter 35: Expedition medicine
Dr Matt Edwards
Specialty Registrar in Emergency Medicine, London School
    of Emergency Medicine;
Faculty, Expedition and Wilderness Medicine courses;
    Ex British Antarctic Medical Officer

Chapter 36: Event medicine
Mr Mark Cutler
Medical Operations Manager,
The Football Association

Chapter 37: Military pre-hospital emergency medicine
Lt Col Jon Walker
Lt Col, RAMC
Consultant in Emergency Medicine
Oxford University Hospitals NHS Foundation Trust

Chapter 38: Careers in pre-hospital emergency medicine
Mrs Joanna Jefferies
Paramedic
Thames Valley Air Ambulance

Abbreviations

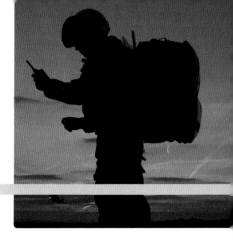

AF	atrial fibrillation
AIM	acute internal medicine
ALS	advanced life support
APS	approved practice settings
AVPU	alert, responsive to voice/pain, unresponsive
BASICS	British Association for Immediate Care
BATLS	battlefield advance trauma life support
BVM	bag-valve-mask (ventilation)
C-spine	cervical spine
CBRN	chemical, biological, radiological, nuclear
CFR	community first responder
CICV	can't intubate, can't ventilate
CPR	cardiopulmonary resuscitation
CSF	cerebrospinal fluid
CT	computed tomography
DCS	damage control surgery
ECRU	enhanced care response unit
EMS	emergency medical services
EPHEC	enhanced pre-hospital emergency care
ETT	endotracheal tube
FAST	focused assessment with sonography in trauma (scan)
FFP	fresh frozen plasma
GCS	Glasgow Coma Scale
GFR	glomerular filtration rate
GMC	General Medical Council
GP	general practitioner
HART	hazardous area response teams
HEMS	helicopter emergency medical service
IBTPHEM	Intercollegiate Board for Training in Pre-Hospital Emergency Medicine
ICH	intracranial haemorrhage
ICM	intensive care medicine
ICP	intracranial pressure
ICS	incident command system
IO	intraosseus

IPPA	inspection, palpation, percussion, auscultation
JESCC	Joint Emergency Services Control Centre
JRCALC	Joint Royal Colleges Ambulance Liaison Committee
LAM	laryngeal mask airway
LPA	lasting power of attorney
MASH	Mobile Army Surgical Hospital
MERT	medical emergency response team
MILS	manual in-line stabilisation
MTC	major trauma centre
NAI	non-accidental injury
NPA	nasopharyngeal airways
OOPE	out-of-programme experience
OPA	oropharyngeal (Guedel) airway
PHEM	pre-hospital emergency medicine
PPE	personal protective equipment
PRU	physician response unit
RCC	rigid cervical collar
ROSC	return of spontaneous circulation
RSI	rapid sequence induction
RT	resuscitative thoracotomy
RTC	road traffic collision
SAD	supraglottic airway device
SBAR	situation, background, assessment, recommendation
SCI	spinal cord injuries
SGSA	Sports Ground Safety Authority
SLUDGE	salivation, lacrimation, urination, defaecation, GI distress, emesis
SOMA	specialist operations medical advisor
STEP	safety triggers for emergency personnel
TARN	Trauma Audit and Research Network
TBI	traumatic brain injury
TCA	traumatic cardiac arrest
TPx	tension pneumothorax
WHO	World Health Organization
WTE	whole-time equivalent

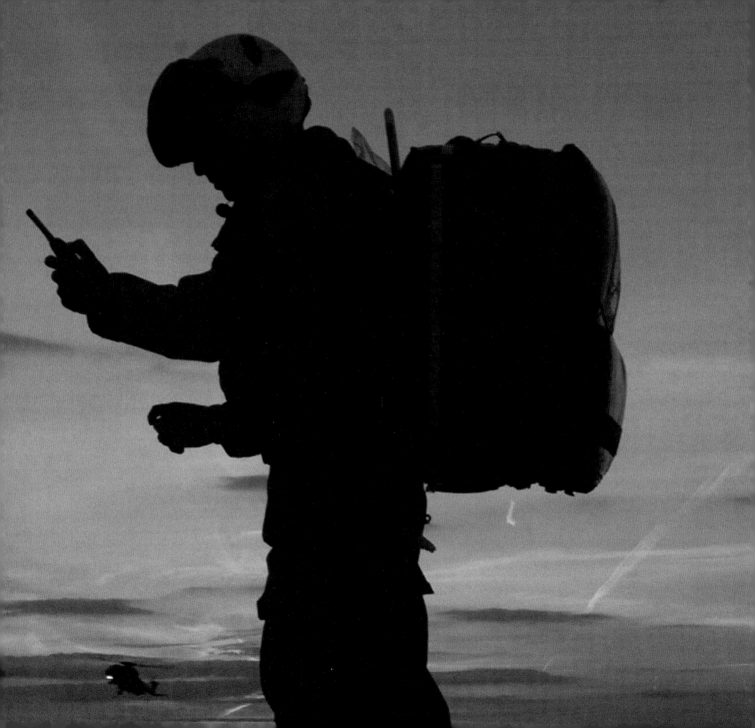

Principles of pre-hospital care

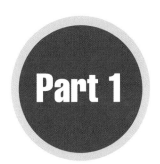

Part 1

Chapters

History of pre-hospital care

Figure 1.1 Pre-hospital care timeline

Biblical	The Good Samaritan
1099	The Knights Hospitaller, the first organised prehospital care service
1797	Jean Larrey's *ambulances volantes*, designed on the battlefields of the Napoleonic War
1869	First civilian ambulance, Bellevue Hospital, NY, USA
1887	St. John's Ambulance founded; first event covered was Queen Victoria's Jubilee
1888	Manchester ship canal: Robert Jones, orthopaedic surgeon, pioneered first comprehensive accident service
1914-18	World War I bore the Thomas splint and the first blood bank
1928	Royal Flying Doctors Service established as the Australian Inland Mission Aerial Medical Service in Cloncurry, Queensland
1956	Peter Safar develops the ABC approach in emergency medicine
1965	The first ever portable defibrillator, installed in Frank Pantridge's Belfast ambulance
1977	BASICS founded by Dr Ken Easton, Yorkshire GP
2013	GoodSAM app launched

Pre-hospital Emergency Medicine at a Glance, First Edition. William Seligman, Sameer Ganatra, Timothy Parker and Syed Masud.
© 2018 John Wiley & Sons, Ltd. Published 2018 by John Wiley & Sons, Ltd.

Pre-hospital emergency medicine (PHEM) is one of the newest specialties in existence, but has a remarkably long history. This chapter chronicles the development of the specialty from ancient times to the modern era, and narrates the evolution of a specialty borne out of necessity, nurtured by enthusiasm, and then ratified by clinical governance.

The beginning

The first insight into pre-hospital care arises from the biblical parable of the Good Samaritan: *'He went to him and bandaged his wounds, pouring on oil and wine. Then he put the man on his own donkey, brought him to an inn and took care of him.'* (Luke 10:34, NIV). From 1500 BC, the invention of the chariot allowed ancient Greeks and Romans to remove injured soldiers from the battlefield, which many regard as the very origin of pre-hospital patient transfer.

The catalyst of war

'War is the only proper school for a surgeon'. These words of Hippocrates embody the truth that war has been the impetus for medical innovation, particularly in trauma, for the past 1000 years. During the crusades, a group of knights set up a hospital for wounded pilgrims in 1023; by 1099, the Order of the Knights Hospitaller had been formed, the first organised, uniformed group providing pre-hospital care. The knights were also known as the Order of St John, and eventually, after a long decline and ensuing revival in the nineteenth century, evolved into the St John's Ambulance we know today.

The eighteenth and nineteenth centuries bore witness to great advances in pre-hospital care through a number of conflicts. Baron Dominique Jean Larrey, surgeon-in-chief of the Napoleonic armies, is credited with instituting the first coordinated pre-hospital care system in 1797, complete with an ambulance service and triage and field hospitals. Impressed by the speed at which the French horse-drawn 'flying artillery' manoeuvred across the battlefield, Larrey developed *ambulances volantes* (flying ambulances), adapting the artillery units and manning them with trained crews. His system of triage was the first to prioritise by clinical need, and not by rank or nationality. The first instance of true aeromedical transportation was documented during the Prussian siege of Paris of 1870 (Franco–Prussian War), in which hot air balloons were used to transport wounded soldiers.

The world wars of the twentieth century catalysed developments, particularly in trauma. The Thomas splint, named after Hugh Owen Thomas, regarded as the father of orthopaedic surgery in the UK, was developed during the First World War and reduced mortality related to compound femoral fractures from 87% to less than 8% over three years. The first blood bank was set up in the First World War and the Second World War saw blood transfusions being performed in the field. The far-reaching nature of the Second World War meant that the front line was often on the streets of London; with ambulance services stretched, the need for doctors on ambulances was questioned for the first time, and this encouraged the development of paramedical services.

In 1942, Igor Sikorsky designed the first mass-producible helicopter, and its potential for rapid evacuation of casualties from the field to treatment areas was swiftly seized upon in later conflicts, especially in Korea and Vietnam. These same wars featured the first mobile army surgical hospital (MASH) units, designed to bring expert surgeons closer to the front lines so that the wounded could be treated more quickly.

War continues to drive innovations in pre-hospital care, with advances in fluid resuscitation, blood transfusion and major haemorrhage control from recent conflicts now being applied routinely by civilian Helicopter Emergency Medical Services (HEMS).

Civilian advances in pre-hospital emergency medicine

The first civilian adoption of military innovations came in the shape of horse-drawn ambulances used in the 1832 London cholera epidemic. Run by the Metropolitan Asylums Board, requests were made by telegram. Ambulance services developed soon after the epidemic, being funded by charities in the UK (e.g. St John's Ambulance) and run by individual hospitals in the USA. The first American ambulance ran from Bellevue Hospital in New York City in 1869. It was manned by an ambulance surgeon equipped with scalpels, saws, splints, laudanum (an opiate) and brandy!

Air ambulances followed. The first known air ambulance was built in North Carolina in 1910; it flew 400 yards before crashing. The Australians then led the world in aeromedical retrieval with the institution of the Royal Flying Doctors Service in 1928. The first air ambulance in the UK launched in Cornwall in 1987 and there are now 27 services operating.

The advent of modern PHEM was heralded by Frank Pantridge, a cardiologist from Belfast. With the ABC algorithm for basic life support having been pioneered by Peter Safar in Pittsburgh, USA, in 1956, Pantridge realised that many patients died from ventricular fibrillation before reaching hospital. As a result, he designed the first portable cardiac defibrillator and fitted it into a van; by 1965, the first mobile coronary cardiac unit was active in Belfast. Over the next few decades, the Belfast treatment system (or 'Pantridge Plan') was adopted by emergency medical services all over the world, and automated external defibrillators were developed for safe use by members of the public.

Pre-hospital emergency medicine in the UK

Pre-hospital care has evolved significantly since the time of Pantridge. It has been transformed over the last four decades from volunteer services (e.g. the British Association for Immediate Care, BASICS) into a recognised subspecialty with a dedicated Faculty and robust clinical governance systems. Volunteers still practise today in the form of community first responders, qualified general practitioners and emergency physicians who give up their time to respond to pre-hospital emergencies.

Further integration between volunteers and structured training programmes is required in the future: such collaboration is intrinsic in order to develop further this life-saving specialty in the UK. Strong governance systems and structure are pivotal for this specialty to continue growing.

Most recently, smartphone applications, e.g. GoodSAM, have been developed that serve to alert trained volunteers to nearby cardiac arrests and other medical emergencies in the community.

Pre-hospital care today

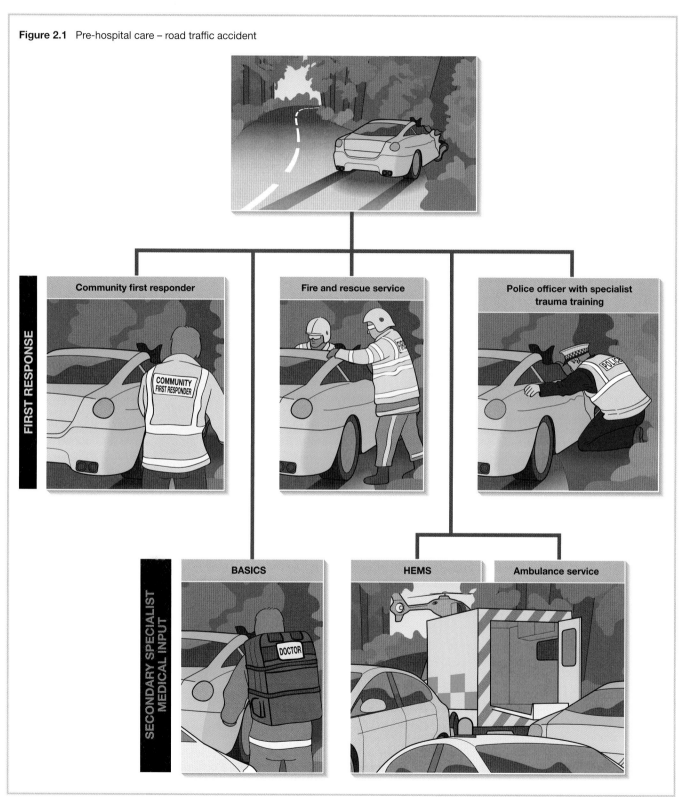

Figure 2.1 Pre-hospital care – road traffic accident

FIRST RESPONSE

Community first responder

Fire and rescue service

Police officer with specialist trauma training

SECONDARY SPECIALIST MEDICAL INPUT

BASICS

HEMS

Ambulance service

Pre-hospital Emergency Medicine at a Glance, First Edition. William Seligman, Sameer Ganatra, Timothy Parker and Syed Masud.
© 2018 John Wiley & Sons, Ltd. Published 2018 by John Wiley & Sons, Ltd.

Pre-hospital care today is an emerging multidisciplinary field. While pre-hospital medical care used to be solely the responsibility of the ambulance service, pre-hospital care today encompasses any specialised medical care delivered outside of the hospital. This care may be provided by first aiders, police officers, fire and rescue services, first responders and physicians, each of whom are trained to varying levels. It is no longer the case that the first medical aid to reach a patient will come from ambulance personnel.

Changes in the ambulance service

Many ambulance services across the UK have now introduced tiered levels of expertise. These will range from volunteer first responder basic aid to advanced paramedics such as the HEMS and critical care-trained paramedics. Advanced/critical care paramedics are trained beyond Joint Royal Colleges Ambulance Liaison Committee (JRCALC) guidelines and are the main providers of enhanced care in the pre-hospital setting. The formation of the physician–paramedic partnership has produced the highest level of enhanced care that the pre-hospital environment can provide.

Hazardous area response teams

Specialist teams, for example Hazardous Area Response Teams (HART), also exist across the UK to provide expertise and support to ambulance crews in a number of different areas. HART has four areas of expertise:

1 Incident response unit – allows HART paramedics to operate inside the inner cordon of a major incident using additional personal protective equipment (PPE) and specialist logistics.
2 Urban search and rescue – allows HART paramedics to deliver care to patients where safe working at height or confined space operations are required.
3 Inland water operations – underwater rescue, e.g. flooding and people injured around rivers or lakes.
4 Tactical medicine operations, e.g. firearms, riots or public disorder, VIP close protection and extraction.

Volunteer first responder schemes

In many cases, volunteers working under the auspices of the local ambulance service may be first on the scene. Community First Responder (CFR) schemes exist across the UK allowing appropriately trained members of local communities to respond to life-threatening emergencies within a short distance of their home or place of work. CFRs are trained to provide basic life support and are used particularly in rural areas where long travel distances delay ambulance response times.

Helicopter emergency medical services

The first air ambulance in the UK began operations in 1987. Now, there are nearly 30 air ambulance charities across the UK flying 20 000 missions per annum. The air ambulance charities in the UK generate over £45 million each year primarily through donations and sponsorship.

Most air ambulances in the UK today carry a physician–paramedic partnership crew and are flown by either one or two experienced specialist pilots. Most HEMS units place one of their specially trained paramedics in the Emergency Operations Centre to monitor incoming calls and the paramedic will then dispatch the duty crew to appropriate incidents. This is often known as a 'dedicated HEMS desk' within ambulance control. Physicians on-board are usually senior trainees or consultants in emergency medicine, anaesthetics or intensive care medicine with additional focused training in PHEM.

Fire and rescue service

In road traffic collisions (RTCs), which account for a significant proportion of trauma seen in the UK, the fire and rescue service may be first on the scene. As well as taking charge of scene safety and extrication of trapped passengers, the fire and rescue services are now able to provide a medical response. Although no national standard exists for medical training in the UK fire service, the majority of fire services now train officers in the following skills:

1 *Airway management*: removal of foreign body; use of suction; jaw thrust; oropharyngeal and nasopharyngeal airways.
2 *Breathing*: use of oxygen; bag-valve-mask ventilation; chest seals; splinting of flail chest.
3 *Circulation*: direct pressure/elevation; tourniquets; basic life support, including automated external defibrillation.
4 *Disability*: assessment of AVPU (alert, responsive to voice/pain, unresponsive).
5 *Spinal management*: manual in-line stabilisation; collar sizing and application; use of spinal board and scoop stretcher; use of Kendrick extrication device.
6 *Burns*: cooling and dressings.

A few ambulance services in the UK are now using fire and rescue services as a primary medical response – this is similar to systems in the USA.

Police

Basic first aid and life support training is provided to all police officers. Advanced medical training is given to specialised subgroups within the police community, including counterterrorism, firearms and close protection units. Specialist units undertake work that may require officers to give medical assistance to the public and to fellow officers at an advanced level, significantly above basic first aid training, e.g. managing ballistic and blast injuries, burns and complex airway issues. Specialist officers will therefore be confident in the use of novel haemostatic agents, chest seals and iGel airways. Police medical training has become significantly more advanced in recent years in response to an increased terrorist threat and the scope of work that has increased for specialist units. A specialist role for doctors within particularly dangerous police operations is rapidly developing. The role of the Specialist Operations Medical Advisor (SOMA) is being recognised more extensively nationally.

Other providers

Other providers of pre-hospital care in the UK include:

• national and international first aid and disaster relief organisations, e.g. Red Cross and St John's Ambulance
• mountain rescue
• Royal National Lifeguard Institution (RNLI)
• cave rescue organisations.

Successful pre-hospital care can only be delivered with effective coordination and management of the attending resources. There is also a need for regular multidisciplinary training scenarios at which all of these different organisations simulate working together on a major incident.

Major trauma pathways in the UK

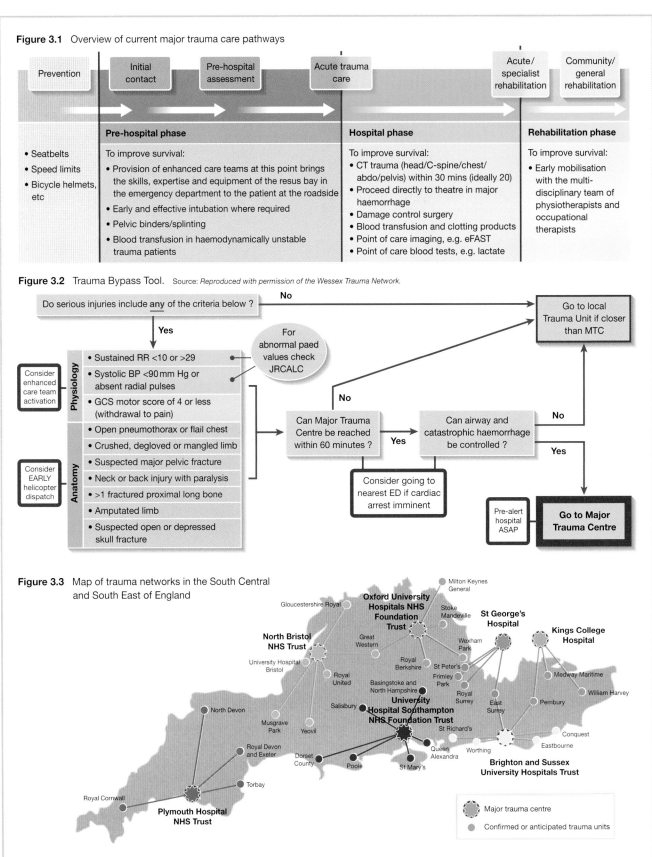

Figure 3.1 Overview of current major trauma care pathways

| Prevention | Initial contact | Pre-hospital assessment | Acute trauma care | Acute/ specialist rehabilitation | Community/ general rehabilitation |

	Pre-hospital phase	**Hospital phase**	**Rehabilitation phase**
• Seatbelts • Speed limits • Bicycle helmets, etc	To improve survival: • Provision of enhanced care teams at this point brings the skills, expertise and equipment of the resus bay in the emergency department to the patient at the roadside • Early and effective intubation where required • Pelvic binders/splinting • Blood transfusion in haemodynamically unstable trauma patients	To improve survival: • CT trauma (head/C-spine/chest/ abdo/pelvis) within 30 mins (ideally 20) • Proceed directly to theatre in major haemorrhage • Damage control surgery • Blood transfusion and clotting products • Point of care imaging, e.g. eFAST • Point of care blood tests, e.g. lactate	To improve survival: • Early mobilisation with the multi-disciplinary team of physiotherapists and occupational therapists

Figure 3.2 Trauma Bypass Tool. Source: Reproduced with permission of the Wessex Trauma Network.

Do serious injuries include any of the criteria below ?

No → Go to local Trauma Unit if closer than MTC

Yes

Consider enhanced care team activation

Physiology
• Sustained RR <10 or >29
• Systolic BP <90 mm Hg or absent radial pulses
• GCS motor score of 4 or less (withdrawal to pain)

For abnormal paed values check JRCALC

Consider EARLY helicopter dispatch

Anatomy
• Open pneumothorax or flail chest
• Crushed, degloved or mangled limb
• Suspected major pelvic fracture
• Neck or back injury with paralysis
• >1 fractured proximal long bone
• Amputated limb
• Suspected open or depressed skull fracture

Can Major Trauma Centre be reached within 60 minutes ?

No →

Yes → **Can airway and catastrophic haemorrhage be controlled ?**

No → Go to local Trauma Unit if closer than MTC

Yes →

Consider going to nearest ED if cardiac arrest imminent

Pre-alert hospital ASAP

Go to Major Trauma Centre

Figure 3.3 Map of trauma networks in the South Central and South East of England

Milton Keynes General
Gloucestershire Royal
Oxford University Hospitals NHS Foundation Trust
Stoke Mandeville
St George's Hospital
Kings College Hospital
North Bristol NHS Trust
Great Western
Wexham Park
University Hospital Bristol
Royal Berkshire
St Peter's
Medway Maritime
Royal United
Basingstoke and North Hampshire
Frimley Park
William Harvey
North Devon
Salisbury
University Hospital Southampton NHS Foundation Trust
Royal Surrey
East Surrey
Pembury
Musgrave Park
Yeovil
St Richard's
Conquest
Royal Devon and Exeter
Dorset County
Poole
Queen Alexandra
Worthing
Eastbourne
St Mary's
Brighton and Sussex University Hospitals Trust
Torbay
Royal Cornwall
Plymouth Hospital NHS Trust

Major trauma centre
Confirmed or anticipated trauma units

Pre-hospital Emergency Medicine at a Glance, First Edition. William Seligman, Sameer Ganatra, Timothy Parker and Syed Masud.
© 2018 John Wiley & Sons, Ltd. Published 2018 by John Wiley & Sons, Ltd.

The burden of trauma

Trauma is the fourth most common cause of death in the western world, and the leading cause of death amongst those aged 1–44 years. The incidence of UK major trauma is estimated at 20 000 cases per annum, with 5400 direct deaths. A further 28 000 cases of serious trauma per annum require major trauma care pathways. The annual cost of trauma treatment is estimated at £0.4 billion, with a concomitant lost economic output of around £3.7 billion (*National Audit Office 2009–2010: Major Trauma Care in England*).

The need for trauma service reform

In 2006, the Royal College of Surgeons published *Provision of Trauma Care*, which found the standard of care in major trauma across the country to be inconsistent, and that UK deaths from major trauma were 40% higher than in the USA. The National Confidential Enquiry into Patient Outcome and Death (NCPOD 2007): *Trauma – Who Cares?* reported that:

- 60% of all trauma cases were managed inadequately
- 40% of all trauma deaths were preventable
- of all hospital trauma calls: 11% did not have a primary survey; 60% received no emergency department consultant review.

The Department of Health's 2008 *Next Stage Review* under Lord Darzi went on to find, 'compelling arguments for saving lives by creating specialised centres for major trauma'. This was echoed by the report from the *National Audit Office 2009–2010: Major Trauma Care in England*:

> Current services for people who suffer major trauma are not good enough. There is unacceptable variation, which means that if you are unlucky enough to have an accident at night or at the weekend, in many areas you are likely to receive worse quality of care and are more likely to die. The Department of Health and the NHS must get a grip on coordinating services through trauma networks, on costs and on information on major trauma care, if they are to prevent unnecessary deaths.
>
> Amyas Morse, Comptroller and Auditor General, NAO

Trauma networks: the new standard of care in major trauma

In *Healthcare for London: A Framework for Action* 2007, Lord Darzi reviewed the available evidence to find that hospitals specialising in major trauma care produced better outcomes; specifically, at the Royal London Hospital, Whitechapel, where a multispecialty trauma service was implemented, mortality rates for major trauma cases in 2006 showed a 26% reduction from the national average. In order to provide a cost-effective service, a network of a smaller number of high-quality trauma specialist hospitals, designated as major trauma centres, was proposed. This was also based on analysis of the system in Quebec, Canada, where implementation of a formalised trauma system, with direct transfer of major trauma patients to specialist trauma centres, resulted in mortality decreasing from 52% to 19%.

In 2009, the Department of Health appointed Professor Keith Willett as National Clinical Director for Trauma Care to oversee and implement the changes proposed by Lord Darzi's *Next Stage Review*. In April 2012, Regional Trauma Networks went live across the country. An independent Trauma Audit and Research Network (TARN) audit found a 20% increase in national major trauma survival rates in the year following the introduction of major trauma networks.

Trauma networks explained

There are now 22 designated major trauma centres (MTCs) nationally. Each MTC provides 24 hour, consultant-led emergency department response and specialist surgical (including cardiothoracic and neurosurgical) services. All patients sustaining major trauma are sent to the nearest designated MTC, even if this is further than another local hospital. Patients are only diverted to specific local hospitals, functioning as trauma units, according to various criteria as determined by the regional trauma service. These typically include situations such as when:

- the patient shows specific physiological signs of instability/anatomical patterns of injury (e.g. airway obstruction) such that they are unlikely to survive primary transfer to an MTC
- the patient is more than 40 minutes away from an MTC.

In these circumstances, trauma units function to stabilise major trauma patients for secondary transfer to the nearest MTC using the minimum possible intervention.

This system means that the most severely injured patients are diverted to MTCs, even if this involves a longer transit time, as direct transfer to an MTC has been shown to reduce mortality and length of stay when compared with secondary transfer.

The need for provision of enhanced pre-hospital emergency care

The 'golden hour' represents a significant window of opportunity for reducing the mortality and morbidity associated with trauma, and is frequently spent outside the hospital environment. Early life-saving interventions, such as resuscitative thoracotomy, require technical expertise and training which typically exceed those of existing paramedic-led emergency medical services (EMS). Skill retention is a further major limitation of the relatively small number of paramedics trained in advanced airway management. Published rapid sequence induction (RSI) and intubation failure rates are significantly higher amongst paramedics than for hospital-trained anaesthetists and emergency medicine trainees. This is unsurprising given that paramedics typically encounter two to three major trauma cases per year and perform three to four intubations, mostly on patients in cardiac arrest. Subspecialty training of hospital doctors in PHEM enables the delivery of emergency department resuscitation bay-level care, at the scene, by practitioners specialising in the regular application of these advanced skills in austere environments.

In 2006, road traffic collisions (RTC) accounted for 3172 deaths and 28 673 serious injuries. In the case of RTCs alone, using published survival rates, physician-led pre-hospital care would save, annually:

- 2041 lives
- £2.6 billion.

Thus, provision of enhanced pre-hospital care is an essential component in improving outcomes in major trauma, and is increasingly recognised as the standard of pre-hospital care in complex polytrauma.

4 Emerging pre-hospital medical care pathways

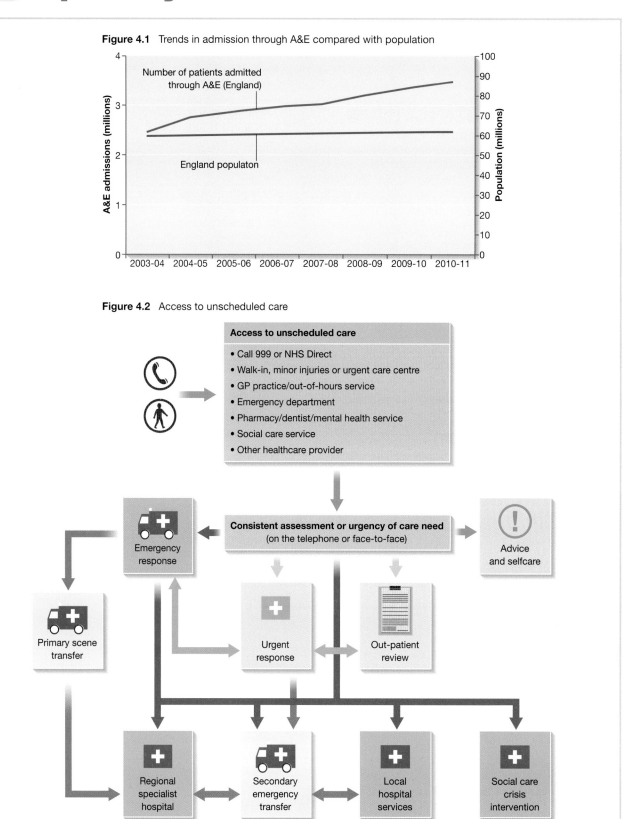

Figure 4.1 Trends in admission through A&E compared with population

Number of patients admitted through A&E (England)

England populaton

Figure 4.2 Access to unscheduled care

Access to unscheduled care

- Call 999 or NHS Direct
- Walk-in, minor injuries or urgent care centre
- GP practice/out-of-hours service
- Emergency department
- Pharmacy/dentist/mental health service
- Social care service
- Other healthcare provider

Emergency response

Consistent assessment or urgency of care need (on the telephone or face-to-face)

Advice and selfcare

Primary scene transfer

Urgent response

Out-patient review

Regional specialist hospital

Secondary emergency transfer

Local hospital services

Social care crisis intervention

Pre-hospital Emergency Medicine at a Glance, First Edition. William Seligman, Sameer Ganatra, Timothy Parker and Syed Masud.
© 2018 John Wiley & Sons, Ltd. Published 2018 by John Wiley & Sons, Ltd.

An increasingly ageing population, representing a progressively more complex patient demographic with multiple medical comorbidities, and public confusion due to a lack of integrated urgent and unscheduled care provision, is placing ever greater pressures on existing urgent and emergency care systems. In light of Professor Keogh's Urgent and Emergency Care Review 2013, and recommendations published as part of the NHS *Five Year Forward View*, it seems likely that restructuring of current pre-hospital emergency care systems will be one part of the solutions required to help meet the changing healthcare demands of the UK population.

The increasing demand for emergency and urgent care services

There were 21.7 million attendances at A&E departments, minor injury units and urgent care centres in 2012/2013, resulting in 5.2 million emergency admissions to England's hospitals in 2012/2013. These figures are steadily increasing (Figure 4.1), representing a huge care burden to the NHS; indeed, urgent and unscheduled care accounts for 100 million NHS contacts each year, corresponding to one-third of all activity and half of all spending.

This increasing burden on urgent care services, combined with public confusion over provision of unscheduled care, is reflected in ever increasing pressures on the ambulance services. Indeed, according to the Health and Social Care Information Centre, in the period 2012/2013 there were 9.08 million emergency calls, an increase of 6.9% from 8.49 million in 2011/2012. Of these calls, 6.98 million (76.9%) resulted in an emergency response arriving at the scene of the incident (cf. 6.71 million, a 4% proportionate increase).

The increasingly complex patient demographic

With life expectancy increasing in the UK, the population age distribution curve is becoming increasingly skewed towards the elderly, with an accordant increase in the number of patients with both chronic disease and multiple comorbidities. Currently, the total number of people with long-term health conditions is estimated at around 15 million; however, the number with three or more conditions is expected to rise from 1.9 million to 2.9 million by 2018.

This ageing demographic is thought to be partly responsible for the increasing pressures on NHS services. The increasing complexity in the treatment requirements of many of these patients makes care by ambulance service personnel, whose function is largely oriented towards the stabilisation of unwell patients for conveyance to hospital, increasingly challenging.

Existing unscheduled care services (Figure 4.2)

Traditional unscheduled care services were provided by general practitioners (GPs), paramedics and emergency departments. As these services struggled to cope with demand, urgent care centres were widely established throughout the UK. However, there is substantial geographical variability in opening hours, walk-in versus referral requirements, and level of service provision such that both the public and healthcare professionals are often uncertain as to what local services are available. Furthermore, urgent care centres have done little to address the needs of the many isolated elderly patients who are unable to arrange their own transport, and are therefore much more likely to call 999 for ambulance support.

The expanding role of physician response units

As the role of the pre-hospital physician has become established in major trauma, the benefits of physician involvement in the pre-hospital environment are becoming more broadly apparent. The additional diagnostic and management capabilities conferred through the presence of a doctor on ambulance call-outs, enables prompt definitive management and significantly aids the decision-making process regarding the need for conveyance to hospital, especially in the context of the complex medical patient with multiple comorbidities.

A retrospective observational study by Bell *et al.* 2006 demonstrated the value of the Physician Response Unit (PRU). Over a 13-month period, the PRU was codispatched as an additional vehicle to emergency calls, meeting the national target 8 minute response time in 82% of cases. Of the 638 patients seen within this period, 39% of patients had medical therapy initiated by the PRU physician, and nearly two-thirds of these had management outside local ambulance protocols. A total of 136 patients (18%) were assessed, treated and prevented from attending the emergency department.

It is likely that PRUs, staffed by experienced PHEM-trained doctors, will play an increasing role in the urgent management of complex medical patients to reduce acute admissions to hospital. More physician-staffed response cars such as the ECRU (Enhanced Care Response Unit) in the Thames Valley are being mirrored throughout the UK. Much of Europe already has a great deal of experience with such systems.

Improving general practice unscheduled care services

In parallel with the above, it is likely that the role of GPs will be modified to provide improved unscheduled care services. Currently, many GP practices opt out of out-of-hours service provision, and batch home visits during working hours to minimise disruption to scheduled GP appointments. A pilot model in St Helens (as referenced in the Keogh Report) provides a dedicated doctor assuming responsibility for all home visits for multiple GP practices within the consortium. Patients are seen within 1 hour of their call, and the visiting doctor has access to their GP records and a direct line to their registered GP. The scheme directly resulted in a 30% decrease in hospital admissions, with a concomitant cost saving of £500 000, thereby demonstrating its cost-effectiveness. It would seem likely that similar schemes are to be more widely adopted.

The shape of the future: integrated urgent and emergency care networks

Professor Keogh's review concluded that, '*Urgent and emergency care networks can improve patient outcomes and experience, however there is variation in the organisation, scope and functionality of networks across the country.*' This has echoes of the findings of the reviews that lead to transformation of UK trauma care, and it seems likely that a similar multifaceted systematic overhaul will be necessary to meet the urgent care demands facing the NHS. The pre-hospital component, delivered by multiple professionals (likely including trained nurses, enhanced care paramedics, GPs and PHEM subspecialty doctors), will be substantial, with emphasis on delivery of enhanced care in patient's homes and integration with existing services to avoid potentially unnecessary hospital admissions. The result will not only be cost savings, but the delivery of expeditious gold-standard patient care at the point of need.

5 Kinematics and mechanism of injury

Figure 5.1 Reading the scene

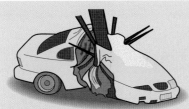

Significant occupant compartment intrusion suggests high energy impact and significant risk of serious injury.

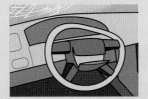

Collision Steering wheel deformation suggests high energy frontal collsion. Suspect serious intrathoracic injuries even in absence of overt signs.

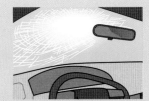

'Bull's eye' fracture of windscreen suggests unrestrained passenger 'up and over' pathway in frontal collision and serious head injury.

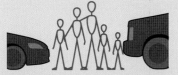

Dent to front of car in vehicle-pedestrian collision; injury from initial impact depends on both the height of victim and the height of the vehicle.

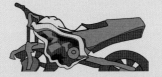

Fuel tank deformation in a motorcycle accident is typically from indentation of the pelvis and predicts severe pelvic injury.

A cracked motorcycle helmet suggests massive energy head impact and the potential for significant head injury

Figure 5.2 Injury pattern prediction in road traffic collisions

Scene signs	Patient signs	Predicted serious injuries
Frontal impact		
'Bull's eye' fracture of windscreen	Craniofacial bruising/lacerations	• Traumatic brain injury • C-spine injury
Deformed steering column	Chest bruising	• Sternal/rib fractures +/− flail chest • Pneumo/haemothorax • Cardiac/pulmonary contusions • Traumatic aortic disruption
Deformed dashboard	Abdominal bruising	• Ruptured spleen, liver, bowel, diaphragm
	Knee bruising/patella dislocation	• Patella fracture • Femoral fracture • Posterior hip dislocation
Lateral impact		
Deformed door with occupant compartment intrusion	Bruised shoulder	• Clavicular fracture • Humeral fracture • Rib fractures (and underlying chest injury)
	Bruised pelvis	• Hip fracture • Pelvic fracture
'B' post deformation	Bruised temple	• Head and C-spine injuries
Rear impact		
Headrest not adjusted		• Whiplash/C-spine hyperextension injuries + any subsequent frontal impact/deceleration injuries
Rotational		
Combination	Combination	• Combination of frontal and lateral impact patterns
Rollover		
Ejection Entrapment		• Multiple and unpredictable injuries, severe • Traumatic amputations/crush syndromes

Figure 5.3 Mechanism of injury

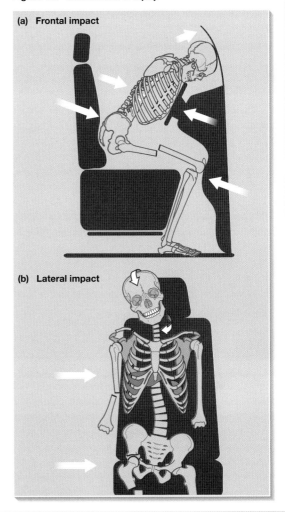

(a) Frontal impact

(b) Lateral impact

Pre-hospital Emergency Medicine at a Glance, First Edition. William Seligman, Sameer Ganatra, Timothy Parker and Syed Masud.
© 2018 John Wiley & Sons, Ltd. Published 2018 by John Wiley & Sons, Ltd.

Energy transfer in trauma

Trauma is tissue disruption that occurs when external energy is transferred to the body at a magnitude and/or rate greater than the ability of the tissue to absorb and dissipate it. The greater the total energy transferred, the greater the damage to the affected tissue. Most trauma results from collisions between two physical bodies, e.g. patient and vehicle or bullet and patient. As kinetic energy = $\frac{1}{2} \times$ mass $\times$ velocity^2, the greatest determinant of kinetic energy transfer is velocity. However, the precise way in which the kinetic energy is transferred to the patient determines the ultimate injury sustained.

The *mechanism of injury* refers to the manner in which trauma has occurred and is pivotal in predicting the likely pattern of injury, e.g. in road traffic collisions or assaults. *Kinematics* refers to the action of forces involved at the time of injury and is useful in the prediction of the type, extent and severity of injury, e.g. a fall from height is much more likely to result in complex polytrauma with immediately life-threatening injuries than a fall from standing.

Reading the scene

In the pre-hospital environment, the witness will often provide only limited and fragmented information. Therefore, careful analysis of the accident site yields many critical clues (Figure 5.1) regarding kinematics and mechanism of injury, which directly influence clinical decision making through prediction of likely patterns of injury. The pre-hospital care practitioner must stop to carefully read the scene to glean as much information as possible. This step is every bit as crucial as the rapid initial ABCDE assessment.

Blunt trauma

Blunt trauma occurs whenever excessive energy transfer causes tissue disruption without skin penetration, as the force is distributed over a relatively large area. Damage is less localised and is caused by temporary cavitation, as the elasticity of the body wall generally causes it to return to its normal shape after the collision. Both direct compression (e.g. lungs compressed between ribs in pulmonary contusion) and shear forces (from differential movement of structures within the body, e.g. sudden deceleration results in forward movement of the aortic arch, while the descending thoracic aorta remains fixed, causing traumatic aortic disruption) contribute to injury. The commonest cause of blunt trauma is RTC, where the 'three collision rule' applies:

1 Initial collision of vehicle with object/vehicle.
2 Collision of passenger with vehicle interior.
3 Collision of passenger's internal organs with other organs/walls of containing compartment.

Reading the scene to establish the velocity and direction of impact (i.e. the kinematics) specific to that particular RTC helps to identify the likely injury patterns, e.g. frontal versus lateral impact.

Penetrating injury

Penetrating injury occurs when an object pierces the skin and enters the tissue of the body to create an open wound or *permanent cavity*. It is classified into ballistic and non-ballistic injury. The external wound bears little or no correlation with either the extent or severity of the internal injury, which must never be underestimated. Urgent CT with/without damage control surgery is the priority in management of these patients, such that scene times must be kept to an absolute minimum.

Ballistic injury

Ballistic injuries are caused by projectiles, typically in the form of either bullets from firearms or shrapnel/fragments from blasts.

Damage is caused by cavitation, both temporary and permanent, the extent of which is determined by the amount of kinetic energy lost by the projectile in the body. This is governed by both *external ballistics,* the behaviour of the projectile from the gun to the target, and *terminal ballistics*, the behaviour of the projectile at the target. The most important external ballistic determinant is projectile muzzle velocity; high velocity rifle rounds (e.g. 7.62 mm or 5.56 mm) typically cause greater penetration and cavitation diameter than lower velocity pistol rounds (e.g. 9 mm or .45 ACP). As projectiles lose their energy over distance, the distance to target is also a key factor.

Terminal ballistic factors affecting cavitation include projectile diameter, deformation (mushrooming), fragmentation and tumble. The internal path of the projectile will determine which specific structures are damaged; however, projectiles will take the path of least resistance through the body and may well ricochet off bony structures to create extensive and convoluted wound tracts. This means that although it is important to look for entry and exit wounds, they may provide misleading information about the internal trajectory of the projectile.

Non-ballistic injury

Non-ballistic penetrating injuries include knife wounds/lacerations, stabbings, piercings and bites. However, shearing, crushing and depth of injury vary considerably according to the weapon used, such that the apparent external injury bears no correlation with the internal injury sustained; this must never be underestimated. For example, the sharpened bicycle spokes/car radio antennae used in gang stabbings create an almost imperceptible external puncture wound yet penetrate into deep tissues and often cause major internal haemorrhage.

Furthermore, in the case of violent assault, patients rarely receive an isolated stab wound, but rather multiple penetrating injuries and potentially additional blunt trauma. Thus, assessment of the patient sustaining non-ballistic penetrating injury differs from the standard primary survey in that it should always begin with 'exposure' in the form of a rapid 'stab check', performed as fast as possible, to check the most vulnerable areas (such as the buttocks) for otherwise occult wounds. This ensures that potentially life-threatening injuries are identified as early as possible, especially in the case of a combative/agitated patient with distracting injury.

Blast injuries

Blast injuries are increasingly encountered both in civilian and military environments due to the increased threat from terrorism and recent conflicts. They are associated with complex polytrauma with multiple mechanisms of injury as described below and should be managed according to the C-ABCDE approach.

1 *Primary blast injuries*: direct barotrauma due to initial blast wave affecting air-filled organs and air–fluid interfaces, e.g. gastrointestinal perforation, alveolar rupture, air embolism, tympanic rupture.
2 *Secondary blast injuries*: trauma due to effects of projectiles (e.g. shrapnel, fragments) transported by the blast wave.
3 *Tertiary blast injuries*: injuries secondary to the initial blast wave, i.e. casualty thrown in the air and then landing against the environment, or fragments of collapsed buildings landing on the patient. Fractures, amputations and head and neck injuries are common, as are secondary complications such as crush and compartment syndrome.
4 *Quaternary blast injuries*: other explosion-related injuries such as burns/toxic inhalations and exacerbations of pre-existing disease, e.g. acute severe asthma.

6 Hazardous materials

Figure 6.1 Hazchem Code.

Source: *Hughes T and Cruickshank J.* Adult Emergency Medicine at a Glance *(2011). Reproduced with permission of John Wiley & Sons.*

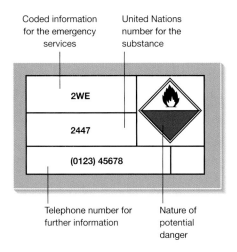

Coded information for the emergency services

United Nations number for the substance

2WE

2447

(0123) 45678

Telephone number for further information

Nature of potential danger

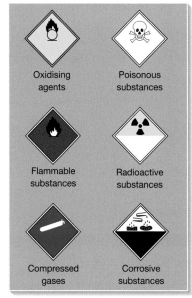

Oxidising agents

Poisonous substances

Flammable substances

Radioactive substances

Compressed gases

Corrosive substances

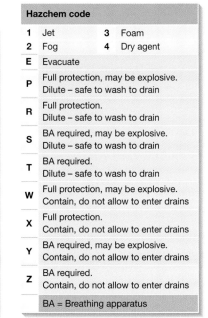

Hazchem code			
1	Jet	**3**	Foam
2	Fog	**4**	Dry agent
E	Evacuate		
P	Full protection, may be explosive. Dilute – safe to wash to drain		
R	Full protection. Dilute – safe to wash to drain		
S	BA required, may be explosive. Dilute – safe to wash to drain		
T	BA required. Dilute – safe to wash to drain		
W	Full protection, may be explosive. Contain, do not allow to enter drains		
X	Full protection. Contain, do not allow to enter drains		
Y	BA required, may be explosive. Contain, do not allow to enter drains		
Z	BA required. Contain, do not allow to enter drains		
	BA = Breathing apparatus		

Figure 6.2 STEP–123 guidance

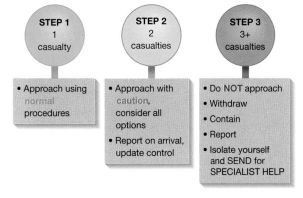

STEP 1 1 casualty
- Approach using normal procedures

STEP 2 2 casualties
- Approach with caution, consider all options
- Report on arrival, update control

STEP 3 3+ casualties
- Do NOT approach
- Withdraw
- Contain
- Report
- Isolate yourself and SEND for SPECIALIST HELP

Figure 6.3 Chemical, biological, radiation and nuclear (CBRN) incident layout

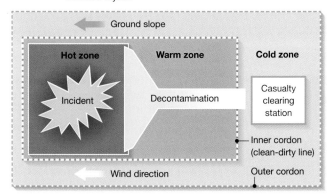

Figure 6.4 Mass decontamination

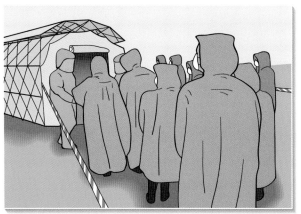

Source: *Figures 6.2, 6.3 and 6.4 redrawn from Nutbeam T and Boylan M.* ABC of Pre-hospital Emergency Medicine *(2013). Reproduced with permission of John Wiley & Sons.*

Hazardous materials are used primarily in industry and research although there is increasing concern over their use in terrorist activities. Exposure to such chemical, biological, radiological and nuclear (CBRN) substances can result in challenging, large-scale medical emergencies. Incidents such as these are within the remit of HARTs, although all responding teams must work together to ensure effective management.

Scene management

Events involving hazardous materials should be approached using an Incident Command System (ICS). The ICS provides a framework to ensure that each responder is informed of their own roles and responsibilities within the operation and contains protocols that are to be followed to coordinate the different teams involved.

Approaching the scene

No pre-hospital care practitioner should approach the CBRN event until after assessment by a HART or other specialist team, for the nature of the toxidrome is seldom initially clear unless a Hazchem code is displayed (Figure 6.1). When on scene, pre-hospital care practitioners should always use the Safety Triggers for Emergency Personnel (STEP) 1-2-3 to guide their approach (Figure 6.2).

There are several difficulties unique to CBRN events which rescuers should bear in mind when assessing the scene (Figure 6.3). CBRN threats may not be easily identifiable by sight, smell or otherwise. Responders should have a low threshold of suspicion for such threats on encountering unusual clinical presentations in multiple patients or after witnessed exposure to unknown chemicals. If exposure is suspected, personnel should not proceed and should remain upwind and uphill of the threat. Defining and containing the scene may be difficult, e.g. in cases of aerosol exposure. Terrorist attacks may feature 'secondary devices' designed to harm rescuers.

Personal protective equipment

Specialised PPE is vital in CBRN events and the exact kit required is determined by the zone in which the rescuer is working and by their level of training. Those in the hot zone, nearest to the source of the exposure, will be HART personnel wearing gas-tight suits and breathing apparatus. Rescuers in the warm zone require chemical-resistant suits with respiratory protection. Those in the cold zone should wear standard PPE including eye protection and a face mask (Figure 6.4).

Decontamination

Once a CBRN event is declared, all patients are considered 'dirty', i.e. contaminated. After decontamination, they become 'clean'. Decontamination is managed by the fire service in partnership with the HART and is usually carried out in dedicated tents set up in the field at a safe distance from the primary event (Figure 6.4). Individuals, including rescuers, are decontaminated using a rinse-wash-rinse protocol:

1 Removal of clothes: the most critical stage of decontamination as clothes may contain up to 90% of the hazardous substance. Clothes are contained in sealed bags and labelled.

2 Rinsing with soapy water to remove surface contaminant and water-based contaminants.

3 Washing with soap and sponges to remove petrochemicals and organic compounds.

4 Rinsing again.

5 Thorough drying and donning clean paper suit.

The water used for decontamination should be collected or directed to storm drains if collection is not possible.

CBRN: specific treatments

There are four main characteristics that determine the overall impact of a hazardous material on a population: toxicity, persistence, latency of action and transmissibility. These features also help with identification of the agent and its specific management.

Chemical agents

There are four main types of chemical agents:

1 *Nerve agents,* e.g. sarin, are anticholinesterase inhibitors, which means that they enhance parasympathetic activity: increased salivation, lacrimation, urination, defaecation, gastrointestinal distress and emesis (SLUDGE) can be caused by moderate exposure, while severe poisoning can cause bronchospasm, respiratory depression, seizures and death. Treatment involves atropine, a muscarinic antagonist, as well as supportive care (ventilation, benzodiazepines for seizures).

2 *Cyanide* binds to mitochondrial cytochromes bringing about a failure of aerobic respiration, rapid circulatory collapse and death. Treatment must be swift. Options include chelation using cobalt EDTA, high-dose hydroxycobalamin or sodium thiosulfate.

3 *Vesicants,* e.g. mustard gas, damage DNA, resulting in the death of exposed tissues: ocular involvement precedes inhalational burns, acute lung injury and skin blistering. Urgent decontamination and burns treatment is indicated.

4 *Pulmonary agents* include phosgene and chlorine. They cause acute lung injury, pulmonary oedema and potentially death. Management is supportive – ventilation and oxygen.

Biological agents

Biological incidents may result from the outbreak of an epidemic (e.g. H5N1 swine 'flu') or biowarfare (e.g. anthrax). Although extremely diverse in terms of presentation, the approach to such events in the pre-hospital environment is generic: supportive care and isolation until specific antidotes can be given in hospital.

Radiological and nuclear agents

Incidents involving radiation exposure include accidents at nuclear power stations and terrorist activity ('dirty bomb': radiological dispersion device). The diagnosis of radiation exposure can be difficult as the lag time between exposure and symptoms varies dramatically. Decontamination is key and dosimeters are used to ensure all radioactive material is removed; note that a patient must be *contaminated* with radioactive material in order to be a threat to others, not merely *exposed* to radiation.

7 Human factors

Figure 7.1 Swiss cheese model. Source: *Reason J. Human error: Models and management. British Medical Journal, 2000:320;768–770. Reproduced with permission of BMJ Publishing Group Ltd.*

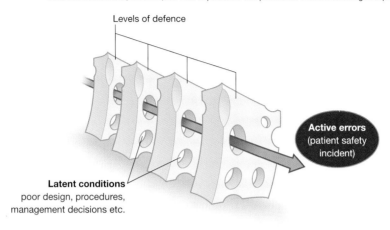

Levels of defence

Active errors
(patient safety
incident)

Latent conditions
poor design, procedures,
management decisions etc.

Figure 7.2 Yerkes-Dodson curve

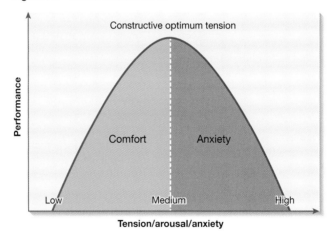

Constructive optimum tension

Performance

Comfort

Anxiety

Low

Medium

High

Tension/arousal/anxiety

Pre-hospital Emergency Medicine at a Glance, First Edition. William Seligman, Sameer Ganatra, Timothy Parker and Syed Masud.
© 2018 John Wiley & Sons, Ltd. Published 2018 by John Wiley & Sons, Ltd.

Pre-hospital emergency medicine takes place within a highly complex and stressful environment where clinicians must make time-critical decisions about unstable patients with incomplete histories working with often unfamiliar teams. These factors render the pre-hospital environment susceptible to error. To minimise the risk of introducing error, the pre-hospital practitioner must have an understanding of how and why mistakes are made as well as an understanding of team resource management. 'Human factors' is defined as enhancing clinical performance through an understanding of the effects of teamwork, tasks, equipment, workspace, culture and organisation on human behaviour and abilities, and the application of that knowledge in clinical settings.

Making mistakes

It is human nature to make mistakes. Whether it is clicking 'send' on an email before double-checking the recipient or getting lost when driving, the consequences can sometimes be serious. However, in healthcare settings, similar types of errors have even greater potential for harmful consequences. The provision of healthcare involves humans working within systems to deliver care. Each system has levels of defence that reduce the chances of making mistakes, e.g. World Health Organization (WHO) surgical checklist. However, these levels of defence have holes – so called 'latent conditions'. This can be represented by the Swiss cheese model in which an ideal system is analogous to a piece of Swiss cheese (Figure 7.1). The holes in the cheese are opportunities for a process to fail and each of the slices is a layer of defence in the process. An error may allow a problem to pass through a hole in one layer but in the next layer the holes are in different places and the problem should be stopped. For a catastrophic error to occur, the holes need to align for each step in the process.

It is uncommon for any single reason or 'failure' to be wholly responsible for an error. Rather, mistakes are typically the result of multiple latent conditions – a series of seemingly minor events that happen consecutively.

Team/crew resource management concepts

There are four key concepts in pre-hospital team resource management which, if all achieved, allow the pre-hospital team leader to get the best out of the pre-hospital team, ultimately leading to the best care for patients.

Bandwidth

Bandwidth is a metaphor that is used to describe the total cognitive processing potential of an individual – the capacity of an individual to perform multiple tasks simultaneously. The Yerkes-Dodson Law suggests that performance increases with psychological or mental arousal, but only up to a point (Figure 7.2). When levels of arousal become too high, when one's bandwidth is full, performance decreases. An early indication of bandwidth saturation is the inability of a person to process new information or take on new tasks. This may be perceived as 'not listening' by those around them. At this point, decision-making is critically impaired. In the pre-hospital environment, tasks should be given to individuals with the greatest free bandwidth and help should be provided to individuals whose bandwidth is likely saturated.

Situational awareness

Situational awareness involves being aware of what is happening around you in order to understand how information, events and your own actions will impact your goals and objectives both now and in the future. In the pre-hospital environment, good situational awareness is achieved by taking a complete overview of the scene, preventing bandwidth saturation and avoiding becoming task-focused. Situational awareness can be enhanced by knowing your team well and encouraging team bonding, sharing information with your team throughout, ensuring that equipment is 'made ready' and checked prior to use and by optimising your physical position such that the whole scene can be seen.

Command gradient

Command gradients are inherent within the medical profession, with a junior doctor unlikely to challenge a professor. There are numerous examples within medical folklore of junior colleagues noticing mistakes as they happen but not speaking up either because they assume their seniors knew what they were doing or for fear of retribution. A flattened hierarchy is therefore an important part of effective team resource management in order to minimise errors. It enables the empowerment of every team member to participate in and question decision making.

Communication

Clear communication is one of the crucial components of safe medical practice. In the pre-hospital environment when working with other emergency service personnel, clear and concise instructions using names can help ensure tasks are completed. Closed-loop communication (asking individuals to report back on the task they have been asked to perform) can be highly effective when the team is large.

8 Pre-hospital transport

Figure 8.1 Thames Valley Enhanced Care Response Unit (ECRU)

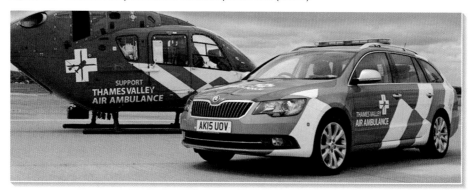

Figure 8.2 Chinook

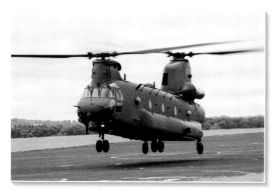

Figure 8.3 Dual-manned ambulance

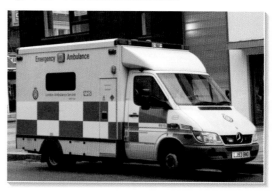

Figure 8.4 KingAir Beechcraft

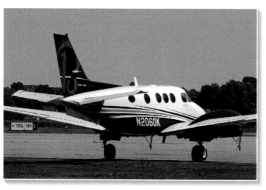

Figure 8.5 RNLI boat

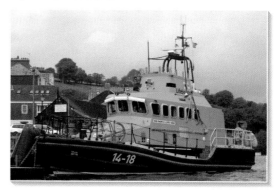

Source: *see reference section.*

Pre-hospital Emergency Medicine at a Glance, First Edition. William Seligman, Sameer Ganatra, Timothy Parker and Syed Masud.
© 2018 John Wiley & Sons, Ltd. Published 2018 by John Wiley & Sons, Ltd.

Unique to the field of pre-hospital care is the need for practitioners to consider how best to get to the incident and how best to get the patient to definitive care. With the range of transport modes at the potential disposal of the pre-hospital care team, it is essential to have a basic understanding of the limitations of each. The decision-making process about the mode of transport is as crucial as the clinical interventions provided to the patient on-scene. Both are integral to the delivery of gold-standard care in the pre-hospital setting. The effects of the mode of transport on the patient, the medical equipment and in limiting possible medical interventions, must all be considered.

Land ambulance

Land ambulances are responsible for the delivery to hospital of the majority of patients in the pre-hospital care setting.

1 Advantages: generally readily available; larger area to work in compared with air transport; easy to pull over if patient deteriorates.
2 Disadvantages: potentially slower than air transport; in spinal injury cases, uneven roads and routes may have a detrimental effect.

Helicopters

Several different types of helicopter are used in UK pre-hospital practice by air ambulance services. The differences between the types of helicopter used are beyond the scope of this text. However, the same principles apply irrespective of which model of helicopter is used.

1 Advantages: short transport times; ability to land in remote environments.
2 Disadvantages: landing sites can be restricted at night-time (only some units in the UK are able to fly at night); difficulty in assessing patients in-flight (noise makes auscultation of chest impossible, for example); unable to fly in adverse weather conditions; unsuitable for transport of certain patient groups, e.g.

psychiatrically unstable; potentially unsafe for unstable patients as able to perform very few interventions in-flight; require regular servicing; some patients have fear of flying; monitoring equipment, e.g. ECG and pulse oximetry affected by heavy vibrations in-flight; may not be possible to land close to the patient – a road vehicle may have better access.

Landing sites

The pilot(s) has the ultimate decision regarding the selection of landing site. Some criteria for the identification of suitable landing sites are listed below:

• a landing site should be twice the diameter of the rotating blades
• the ground must be firm and flat
• the site must be away from power or telephone lines and free of debris
• the site should be clear of people (this may necessitate making several low passes over the landing site with flashing lights in order to encourage people to move away).

Practitioners often use the terms pre-hospital care and HEMS interchangeably. However, it must be appreciated that although helicopter transport plays an integral role in delivery of enhanced care at the scene, it also has significant limitations that the pre-hospital care practitioner must be aware of. The PHEM practitioner must understand, appreciate and consider all other modes of transport.

Fixed wing aircraft

Fixed wing aeromedical retrieval is uncommon in UK pre-hospital care practice. The main advantage of a fixed wing aircraft over a helicopter is the distance it is able to travel. With the UK being geographically much smaller than countries such as Australia or the USA, the disadvantage of fixed wing aircraft – that they require an airfield to land – significantly outweighs the benefit. Around the world, however, fixed wing aircraft are being used regularly for retrieval.

9 Scene safety

Figure 9.1 HEMS kit

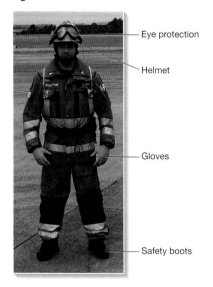

- Eye protection
- Helmet
- Gloves
- Safety boots

Figure 9.2 Specialist equipment

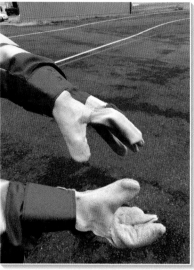

(a) Extrication gloves

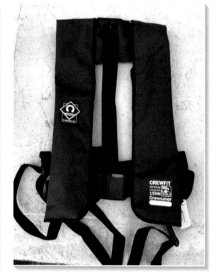

(b) Personal flotation device

Figure 9.3 Example of scene safety – derailed cargo train

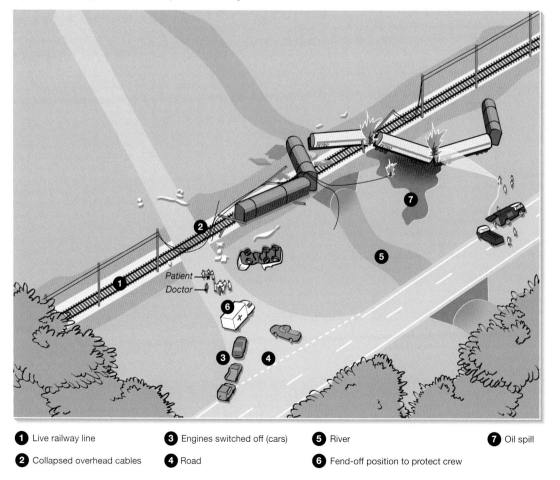

Patient
Doctor

1 Live railway line   **3** Engines switched off (cars)   **5** River   **7** Oil spill

2 Collapsed overhead cables   **4** Road   **6** Fend-off position to protect crew

Pre-hospital Emergency Medicine at a Glance, First Edition. William Seligman, Sameer Ganatra, Timothy Parker and Syed Masud.

Importance of scene safety

The mantra at the forefront of the mind of any pre-hospital care practitioner has always been: is it safe to approach? Although scene control is primarily the responsibility of the fire and police crews, it is no help to the casualty or the other rescuers if any harm comes to the medics, and so every practitioner must be personally vigilant for hazards. Always think of your own safety first, then the safety of other rescuers and bystanders, and finally the safety of the patient. This is the 1-2-3 of safety.

Initial approach and arrival at the scene

On arriving at the scene, assess it thoroughly for hazards to your team and to other rescuers. One should communicate with crew members already on the scene to obtain as much information about current and former dangers. If the scene has not yet been made safe, then this should be left to the fire and police crews. It is vital to understand that the scene is a *dynamic* environment. Factors in scene safety may include the following: cutting of vehicles, movement of power cables, leaking fuel and live rail tracks. What was once judged to be safe may become decidedly – and sometimes unpredictably – unsafe. Assessment of scene safety is a dynamic process.

Personal protective equipment (Figures 9.1–9.2)

Pre-hospital care practitioners have to be able to work in a diverse range of environments, from the roadside, to water, to areas with chemical or nuclear hazards. As a result, rescuers are exposed to risks from multiple sources, and so require a full range of PPE and the training to use it effectively:

1 *Helmet* with adjustable headband and strap to prevent practitioners from removing a loose helmet that obscures their view when bending over to treat a patient.
2 *Eye protection* from debris as well as from splashes of bodily fluids, especially patient blood: assume that all patients are positive for bloodborne viruses.
3 *Ear protection* is essential in noisy environments: ear defenders or earplugs.
4 *Facemasks* are used to prevent the inhalation of debris and specialised masks, e.g. the FFP3 mask, have additional filters to stop the transmission of airborne pathogens, e.g. tuberculosis and influenza.
5 *Gloves*, as in the hospital environment, are indispensible in preventing transmission of infection; alcohol gel should be used before and after donning gloves. Heavy-duty extrication gloves must be worn when operating around exposed sharp edges and hot surfaces.
6 A *high visibility jacket* is mandatory for working on or near roads and for low-visibility settings.
7 Robust *safety boots* with a reinforced toecap must be worn to ensure crewmembers can move around the scene unimpeded by terrain or debris.

Special considerations

The above principles of scene safety should be applied universally in the pre-hospital environment. However, we will now discuss specific measures that should be taken in several commonly encountered scenarios.

Road traffic collisions

Attending road traffic collisions is dangerous due to risks from passing traffic and damaged vehicles. The first emergency vehicle on scene should adopt the 'fend-off position', where the vehicle is parked diagonally across the blocked lane, acting as a barrier between oncoming traffic and the treatment area. By parking diagonally, if the ambulance is shunted by a passing car, it will not be pushed forward into the casualty and crew. Traffic cones should also be used to cordon off the area as efficiently as possible and roads closed where necessary. All emergency vehicles should be stabilised with handbrakes and chocks applied, and engines switched off. Appropriate warning signs should be used to warn oncoming motorists of an incident ahead. Communication with the fire service is paramount here: ensure that any fuel leakages are cleared and be aware of warnings given by the fire service during extrication. Be wary of any hazardous cargo and alert the fire service or hazardous materials personnel if necessary. Look for any undeployed devices, e.g. airbags and seatbelt pretensioners, and remain clear of them where possible; apply restraints if required.

Railways

Ensure that power to overhead cables or to live rail has been isolated and switched off. Remember that diesel trains are still able to run without electricity (see Figure 6.3).

Water

The risk of becoming a casualty oneself during a water rescue is high. Crews must undergo specialist training and be equipped with the specialist kit required for water, e.g. lifejackets; these inflate automatically upon contact with water. Water rescue should not be attempted by non-specialist teams.

Fire

Scenes involving fire must always be tackled by the fire service in the first instance, and all crews must act under their guidance. In terms of PPE, fire-retardant suits made of Nomex or Kermel fibres are required, and full-length cotton undergarments are recommended to keep the underlying skin as cool as possible. All HEMS crewmembers are required to wear flame-retardant flight suits due to possible exposure to aviation fuel (Figure 9.1).

Electrical incidents

As stated above, the medical team should take responsibility for its own safety. The clear risk is of further electrocution and so ensure that the electricity supply is switched off before approaching the scene – check this yourself. Consider nominating a police officer to supervise the switch to guarantee that the supply remains turned off while on the scene. Be aware of any electrical conductors nearby, e.g. water, and clear them before embarking on treatment. The type of current (alternating or direct) is important in directing management: AC (domestic, railway) tends to cause ventricular fibrillation, while large DC (industrial, lightning, railway) shocks can cause asystole. Industrial guidelines state that personnel should stay 3 m away from 750 V–150 kV cables, 4.5 m from 151 kV–250 kV cables, and at least 6 m from cables of higher voltages.

You are ultimately responsible for your own safety; reassess hazards continually.

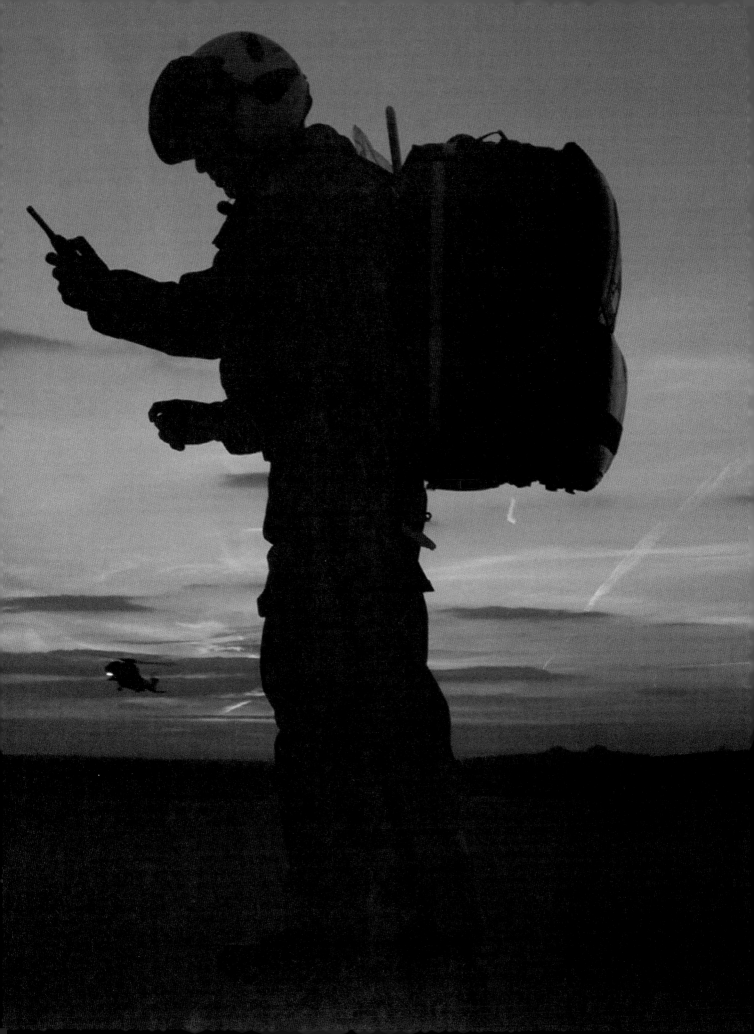

Initial assessment and management of immediately life-threatening injuries

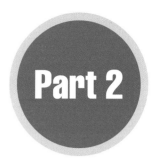

Part 2

Chapters

10 The primary survey

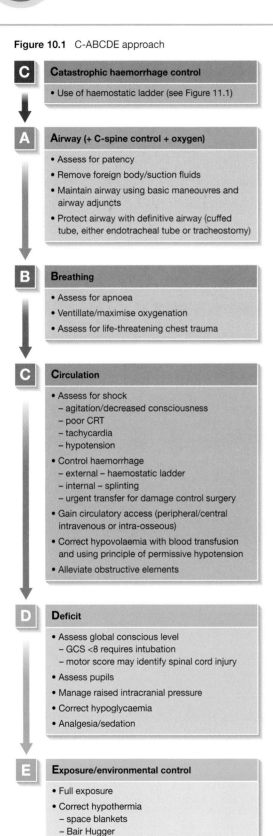

Figure 10.1 C-ABCDE approach

C | Catastrophic haemorrhage control
- Use of haemostatic ladder (see Figure 11.1)

A | Airway (+ C-spine control + oxygen)
- Assess for patency
- Remove foreign body/suction fluids
- Maintain airway using basic maneouvres and airway adjuncts
- Protect airway with definitive airway (cuffed tube, either endotracheal tube or tracheostomy)

B | Breathing
- Assess for apnoea
- Ventilate/maximise oxygenation
- Assess for life-threatening chest trauma

C | Circulation
- Assess for shock
  - agitation/decreased consciousness
  - poor CRT
  - tachycardia
  - hypotension
- Control haemorrhage
  - external – haemostatic ladder
  - internal – splinting
  - urgent transfer for damage control surgery
- Gain circulatory access (peripheral/central intravenous or intra-osseous)
- Correct hypovolaemia with blood transfusion and using principle of permissive hypotension
- Alleviate obstructive elements

D | Deficit
- Assess global conscious level
  - GCS <8 requires intubation
  - motor score may identify spinal cord injury
- Assess pupils
- Manage raised intracranial pressure
- Correct hypoglycaemia
- Analgesia/sedation

E | Exposure/environmental control
- Full exposure
- Correct hypothermia
  - space blankets
  - Bair Hugger

Table 10.1 Glasgow Coma Scale. *Source: Adapted from http://www.glasgowcomascale.org/*

Behaviour	Response	Score
Eye opening	Spontaneous	4
	To speech	3
	To pain	2
	No response	1
Best response: verbal	Fully oriented	5
	Confused speech	4
	Inappropriate words	3
	Incomprehensible sounds	2
	No response	1
Best response: motor	Obeys commands	6
	Localises to painful stimulus	5
	Withdraws from painful stimulus	4
	Flexes to pain (decorticate)	3
	Extends to pain (decerebrate)	2
	No response	1
Severity of TBI	Minor brain injury	13–15
	Moderate brain injury	9–12
	Severe brain injury	3–8

Principles of rapid initial assessment

The primary survey forms the rapid initial assessment of the acutely unwell patient in any context, and in the case of major trauma is directed exclusively at identifying and treating immediately life-threatening injuries. The systematic, stepwise approach of C-ABCDE (Figure 10.1) ensures that pathology is addressed in the order of speed of fatality; airway compromise will kill more quickly than hypoglycaemia. Equally as important is the need to reassess the patient constantly from the beginning each time an intervention is made, as pathology rapidly evolves. Initial assessment is a repeated dynamic process.

As ever in the pre-hospital phase, the clinician will already have a good idea of the likely pathology and provisional management plan before even reaching the patient, based on information gleaned from the initial callout history and reading the scene on arrival.

Catastrophic haemorrhage

Increasing experience of major trauma in combat has led to the recognition that even before airway obstruction, catastrophic external arterial bleeding will lead to rapid exsanguination and death. This is particularly common in traumatic limb amputation, where arteries are often incompletely transected and hence unable to fully retract and constrict to limit haemorrhage. The ladder approach to significant bleeding enables rapid haemostatic control.

Airway (+ cervical spine control + oxygen)

If the patient is talking, the airway is presumed clear. If the patient is not talking, look, listen and feel for breathing while simultaneously feeling for a central pulse. If the patient is not breathing and a pulse is absent, manage cardiac arrest according

Pre-hospital Emergency Medicine at a Glance, First Edition. William Seligman, Sameer Ganatra, Timothy Parker and Syed Masud.
© 2018 John Wiley & Sons, Ltd. Published 2018 by John Wiley & Sons, Ltd.

to cause. If the patient is not breathing, open the mouth and look for obvious causes of upper airway obstruction, e.g. foreign body (remove if easily accessible), vomitus/blood (suction). Additional sounds such as snoring imply partial upper airway obstruction due to loss of oropharyngeal tone and can be managed using the airway management ladder (manoeuvres/adjuncts/supraglottic devices/definitive airway); stridor, indicating distal upper airway obstruction, and significant orofacial trauma/inhalational injury may require a surgical airway. Manual in-line stabilisation of the cervical spine (C-spine) is of paramount importance to reduce risk of further damage/death from potential unstable C-spine fracture and goes hand-in-hand with assessment of the airway. After securing the airway, all patients must receive high flow oxygen to maximise oxygenation and minimise tissue hypoxia.

The C-spine is typically secured with three-point immobilisation. At the same time, all monitoring should be applied to the patient. The neck is then quickly examined for distended neck veins (obstructive shock), tracheal deviation (mediastinal shift), surgical emphysema (pneuomothorax/upper airway disruption) and distorted surface anatomy (laryngeal disruption).

Breathing

Once the airway is secured, breathing is assessed using IPPA (inspection, palpation, percussion, auscultation). The first priority is identification of apnoea; patients not spontaneously breathing or with inadequate respiratory rate (fewer than eight breaths per minute) require ventilation. This is often initially with bag-valve-mask; the disadvantage is that this introduces large volumes of air into the stomach, with distension and subsequent vomiting which compromise the airway. Intubation is therefore the management of choice.

Further assessment of breathing is aimed at identification of immediately life-threatening chest pathology (Table 10.2).

Circulation

Haemorrhage is the predominant preventable cause of death following major trauma. The patient is assessed for signs

Table 10.2 Immediately life-threatening chest pathology

Condition	Findings (affected side)	Management
Tension pneumothorax	Asymmetrical chest movement Hyper-resonance Absent breath sounds	Needle decompression and thoracostomy
Open chest wound	Bubbling blood from open chest defect	Three-sided occlusive dressing
Massive haemothorax	Asymmetrical chest movement Dullness to percussion Absent breath sounds	Good vascular access, thoracostomy
Flail chest	Paradoxical chest wall segment movement	Good analgesia/ intubation and ventilation if respiratory compromise

Table 10.3 Sites of major internal haemorrhage

Site	Example injury	Specific management
Chest	Pulmonary artery dissection causing massive haemothorax	Tube thoracostomy/ resuscitative thoracostomy with lobar compression
Abdomen	Splenic rupture, liver laceration	REBOA*/urgent transfer for damage control surgery
Pelvis	Open book pelvic fracture	Pelvic binder
Long bones	Femoral shaft fracture	Fracture reduction and traction splint

*Resuscitative endovascular balloon occlusion of the aorta

of circulatory shock, with general management directed at haemostasis, gaining circulatory access for correction of hypovolaemia and alleviation of any obstructive elements of shock.

Life-threatening haemorrhage with hypovolaemic shock occurs in five sites, often remembered as 'blood on the floor and four more,' to ensure that occult internal bleeding is not overlooked. External haemorrhage is managed using the haemostatic ladder (see Chapter 11). Of particular note, craniofacial injuries with apparently superficial bleeding will lose large volumes of blood insidiously as the tight fascia restricts vasospasm of lacerated arteries and veins (Table 10.3).

Obstructive shock may be due to impaired venous return from massive haemothorax/tension pneumothorax (which should already have been identified and managed in the assessment of breathing), or from cardiac tamponade following penetrating thoracic injury, which will require resuscitative thoracotomy.

Deficit (neurology)

Determining the patient's neurological status is of significant importance. Global conscious level is rapidly assessed using the AVPU score (alert, responsive to voice/pain, or unresponsive). Once time allows, a patient's neurological status can be assessed more precisely with the Glasgow Coma Scale (GCS) (Table 10.1).

A GCS <8 correlates with an AVPU score of pain and is associated with loss of protective airway reflexes, potentially requiring a definitive airway. The motor score may elicit localising signs suggesting spinal cord injury. Pupils should be assessed for size and reactivity to light; asymmetry may be indicative of raised intracranial pressure, e.g. due to evolving intracranial haemorrhage. Both may necessitate an urgent transfer to a neurosurgical centre. Glucose should be measured and hypoglycaemia corrected as it is rapidly fatal and may have precipitated the initial injury.

Exposure and environmental control

Temperature should be measured and patients warmed with blankets to help reverse hypothermia, one of the components of the 'lethal triad' in trauma (see Chapter 11). Full exposure at each stage of assessment facilitates rapid identification of life-threatening injuries, but risks contributing to lower body temperature with its consequent effects.

11 Control of major haemorrhage

Figure 11.1 Mechanism of lethal triad. Source: *http://www.open.edu/openlearn/health-sports-psychology/health/public-health/understanding-the-bodys-response-injury-and-the-development-trauma-centres (accessed November 2016). Reproduced with permission of The Open University.*

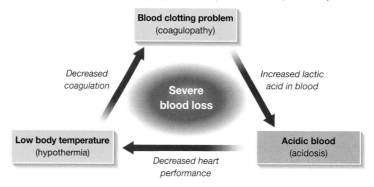

Figure 11.2 Haemostatic ladder

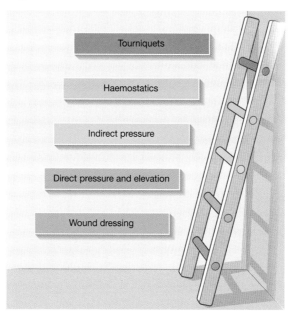

Figure 11.3 Systemic anticoagulation

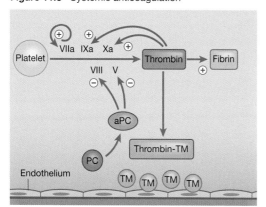

Abbrev: aPC, activated protein C; PC, protein C; TM, thrombomodulin

Figure 11.4 Increased fibrin breakdown

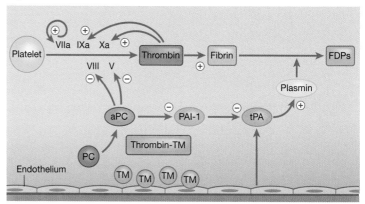

Abbrev: PAI-1, plasminogen activator inhibitor-1; tPA, tissue plasminogen activator

Pre-hospital Emergency Medicine at a Glance, First Edition. William Seligman, Sameer Ganatra, Timothy Parker and Syed Masud.
© 2018 John Wiley & Sons, Ltd. Published 2018 by John Wiley & Sons, Ltd.

The problem of major haemorrhage in trauma

Uncontrolled haemorrhage has been shown to be the most common cause of preventable deaths in trauma and is responsible for 40% of early in-hospital trauma mortality. Observational studies have shown that 25% of trauma patients also have an established coagulopathy on arrival in the emergency department and that this is associated with a fourfold increase in mortality.

The so-called 'lethal triad of death' (Figure 11.1) describes the mutually perpetuating combination of acute coagulopathy, hypothermia and metabolic acidosis. These are seen in exsanguinating trauma patients. Hypoperfusion results in reduced oxygen delivery and the consequent switch to anaerobic metabolism results in lactate production and therefore metabolic acidosis. Anaerobic metabolism limits heat production, exacerbating hypothermia caused by exposure to cold resuscitation fluids and blood.

Acute coagulopathy in trauma

It is known that disruption of haemostatic equilibrium occurs at the moment of traumatic impact at which point physiological responses are initiated producing acute traumatic coagulopathy. The degree of coagulopathy has been shown to correlate closely with severity of injury, blood product requirements and mortality. Although the aetiology of acute coagulopathy in trauma is not fully understood, it is thought to involve the disruption of the equilibrium of the clotting cascade:

- procoagulant impairment: fibrinogen has recently been identified as an important mediator in acute coagulopathy in trauma with levels falling early in major haemorrhage. As fibrinogen has an essential role to play in effective clot formation, supplementation is being investigated as a therapeutic option in major haemorrhage
- systemic anticoagulation (e.g. via activation of protein C secondary to tissue hypoperfusion)
- increased fibrin breakdown: tranexamic acid (an inhibitor of fibrinolysis) should be administered pre-hospital in patients with major haemorrhage
- platelet dysfunction
- endothelial activation: leading to increased fibrin breakdown as well as inactivating procoagulant factors.

The ladder approach to pre-hospital haemorrhage control

Under normal circumstances, major external haemorrhage may be controlled by the stepwise application of basic techniques – the so-called haemostatic ladder (Figure 11.2). The first step on the ladder is a basic wound dressing. This should be applied together with direct pressure and elevation. Should these techniques fail, haemostatic dressings may be applied, particularly in junctional zones, e.g. neck, axilla, groin, perineum, where the application of a tourniquet would be impractical. These contain factors that promote coagulation by attracting red cells or concentrating coagulation factors. Tourniquets may also be used if blood loss cannot be controlled using other means. They should be placed as distally as possible on the injured limb and should be tightened until the bleeding ceases. Adequate analgesia is essential when applying an arterial tourniquet.

Bleeding within the thoracic cavity will be very difficult to manage without enhanced care. Bleeding within this area may require specifically the advanced technique of thoracotomy which will confer the ability to stop vessel and organ damage that is causing bleeding (and may compromise ventilation and oxygenation, in which case thoracostomy should be performed in the pre-hospital setting). Bleeding into the pericardium should be controlled before hospital by thoracotomy and repair of damaged myocardium, and clots evacuated. All other bleeding into the thorax or abdomen must be controlled operatively and therefore early disposition is recommended.

Long bone fractures can bleed significantly and must be drawn out to length and splinted in position to prevent further bleeding

Damage control resuscitation

While pre-hospital teams are vital in the initial management of major haemorrhage, surgery is the definitive intervention in the context of severe blood loss and scene times must therefore be limited. The concept of 'damage control resuscitation' has emerged in recent years. It involves the following key components:

- *Haemostatic resuscitation*: this describes the very early use of blood and blood products as primary resuscitation fluids.
- *Permissive hypotension*: this is a relatively new concept whereby the target blood pressure is set as low as is necessary to ensure adequate organ perfusion, but no higher. Higher blood pressures are associated with haemodilution and clot disruption. Target systolic pressure is 80–100 mmHg (radial pulse should be palpable).
- *Damage control surgery*: this is the definitive way of controlling major haemorrhage and is surgery limited to what is needed to control haemorrhage. Pre-hospital efforts should be focused on limiting time delays on-scene to allow rapid transport to hospital for definitive surgical intervention once the patient has sufficient physiological reserve.

12 Cervical spine injuries

Box 12.1 The Nexus low-risk criteria

> **Cervical spine radiography is indicated for patients with trauma unless they meet all of the following criteria:**
>
> - No posterior midline cervical spine tenderness
> - No evidence of intoxication
> - A normal level of alertness
> - No focal neurologic deficit
> - No painful distracting injuries

Figure 12.1 The Canadian C-spine rule   Source: *Hofmann, et al. (1998). Reproduced with permission of Elsevier.*

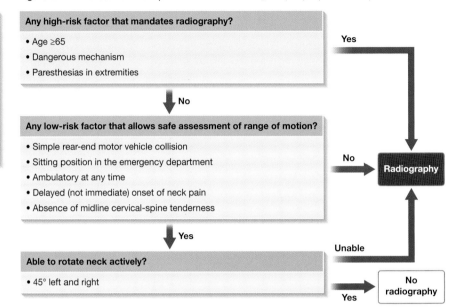

Any high-risk factor that mandates radiography?

- Age ≥65
- Dangerous mechanism
- Paresthesias in extremities

— No →

Any low-risk factor that allows safe assessment of range of motion?

- Simple rear-end motor vehicle collision
- Sitting position in the emergency department
- Ambulatory at any time
- Delayed (not immediate) onset of neck pain
- Absence of midline cervical-spine tenderness

— Yes →

Able to rotate neck actively?

- 45° left and right

Yes → Radiography

No → Radiography

Unable → Radiography

Yes → No radiography

Figure 12.2 Safe helmet removal

Motorcyclists are at high risk of suffering from C-spine injuries. This is due to the high-speed nature of collisions as well as the lack of a car's protective crumple zone. Modern motorcycle helmet design has enhanced head and neck protection during impact, but helmet removal by the prehospital care team carries its own risk of damaging the C-spine due to the mobilisation required.

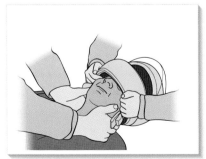

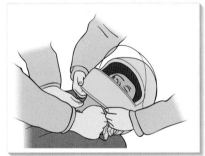

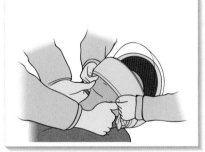

1. Two pre-hospital practitioners trained in safe helmet removal are required for the procedure. The first clinician should position themselves at the head end of the patient and provide manual in-line stabilisation (MILS). The second clinician should release or cut chin straps and guards.

2. The second clinician now carefully takes over the provision of MILS from the caudal end of the patient. The first clinician gently flexes the helmet apart laterally and removes it in a steady motion, avoiding movement of the neck.

3. As the helmet is being removed by the first clinician, the second clinician continues to provide MILS by placing their thumbs on the mandible and by supporting the occiput with the rest of their hands.

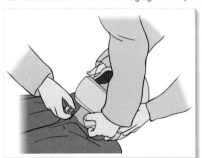

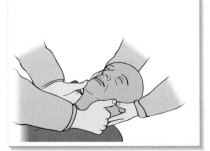

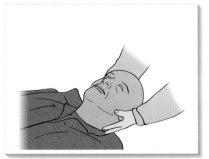

4. If the helmet covers the entire face, the nose may impede removal. To clear the nose, tilt the helmet backward to raise it over the nose.

5. Ensure that the weight of the patient's head is supported throughout the process of helmet removal.

6. MILS is once again provided from the head end of the patient by clinician 1 until three-point immobilisation is established.

Pre-hospital Emergency Medicine at a Glance, First Edition. William Seligman, Sameer Ganatra, Timothy Parker and Syed Masud.
© 2018 John Wiley & Sons, Ltd. Published 2018 by John Wiley & Sons, Ltd.

Spinal cord injury most commonly affects the extremes of age, i.e. the young and the elderly, and its effects can be life-long. Trauma-related spinal cord injuries affect between 280 and 320 people in every million in Western Europe, and 25–50% of those involve the cervical spinal cord. Patients with C-spine injuries have the highest reported early mortality rate in spinal trauma as, owing to the anatomy, trauma to this section of the spine commonly causes cord damage. Prompt spinal immobilisation and detection of these injuries is paramount in avoiding additional spinal cord injury.

There are seven cervical vertebrae which enclose the spinal cord in the neck. It is the same anatomical arrangement that allows us to flex, extend, and rotate our neck that gives rise to cervical cord injuries in trauma: cord damage tends to occur at the junction of the mobile C-spine and the relatively fixed thoracic spine (C5, C6, C7 and T1). Fractures of the odontoid peg of C2 are also extremely common. Four key mechanisms of injury – often in combination – are responsible: hyperflexion, hyperextension, rotation and compression of the spine. Half of all C-spine injuries follow road traffic accidents, in which these four mechanisms are often involved.

Identifying cervical spine injury

Casualties with C-spine injuries are a high-risk group, and damage to the high cervical spine may even prove immediately fatal due to paralysis of the muscles of respiration. Most cases of cord injury are partial, affecting solely individual motor or sensory tracts, resulting in varying degrees of disability. It is now recognised that in an increasing proportion of cases, considerable neurological recovery is possible, provided that the injured C-spine is managed appropriately. The spinal canal is relatively wide within the C-spine, and so the cord has room to move and hence undergo further damage from unstable axial fractures. As a result, effective spinal immobilisation can prevent any further injury and optimise spinal recovery. Therefore, it is imperative to rapidly identify C-spine injury on approaching the scene of any trauma patient.

Assessing the cervical spine

Manual immobilisation of the C-spine should be commenced immediately in *all* trauma patients while the initial assessment is undertaken.

History

The mechanism of injury is important in determining whether spinal cord injury is likely to have occurred as well as the nature of the damage. Road traffic accidents, falls, and sporting injuries are responsible for most C-spine fractures, and the mechanism can often be deduced from the incident, e.g. hyperextension and then hyperflexion in rapid deceleration collisions. The patient may also report midline spinal pain.

Examination

C-spine tenderness can be elicited by palpating the back of the neck in the midline, while maintaining manual immobilisation. A rapid assessment of movement and sensation in all four limbs should also be carried out during the primary survey.

Cervical spine clearance

Identification and assessment of C-spine injury in the field may be challenging if patients present with a reduced GCS. This may be because of concomitant head injury or intoxication (alcohol, sedative or analgesic medication). Furthermore, high levels of circulating catecholamines and endogenous opioids in trauma patients conspire to mask spinal fractures. C-spine immobilisation can often make it more difficult to deliver certain interventions (e.g. endotracheal intubation), and in some situations cause direct harm to the patient. Clinical decision rules have thus been formulated to guide the practitioner as to when C-spine immobilisation can be safely discontinued. The NEXUS guidelines and Canadian C-Spine Rule (Box 12.1 and Figure 12.1) both have a high sensitivity but low specificity. This means that they can be used safely to rule out significant C-spine injury and allow appropriate spinal immobilisation. Initially used in the emergency department as a means to clear patients with suspected spinal injury without radiological assessment, these guidelines are also used reliably in the pre-hospital environment.

It is important to remember, however, that spinal immobilisation, and *not* spinal clearance, is the priority in multiple trauma.

Securing the cervical spine

The principle of minimal movement, maximum safety applies to all spinal injuries. The use of a scoop stretcher, the practice of scoop-to-skin immobilisation and 10° tilts all minimise further spinal cord damage. As well as these, there are specific measures to stabilise the C-spine:

1 *Manual in-line stabilisation (MILS)* is performed on an upright or supine patient. The practitioner stands behind or above the patient and holds the patient's head in a neutral position while locking their own elbows or resting them on the ground to stabilise them. This should prevent any side-to-side head movement. Two centimetres of padding placed under the head in healthy, supine patients can optimise the neutral position of the head relative to the body. MILS should be initiated immediately on reaching the patient.

2 *Rigid cervical collars (RCCs)* reduce C-spine movement by 80–90% but only when used in combination with blocks and tape; MILS should be performed until such 'three-point immobilisation' is applied. C-spine mobility is reduced by 90-95% when three point immobilisation is used with an extrication device or a spinal board.

Caveats in immobilisation

There are some situations in which the risks of MILS and RCC can outweigh the benefits:

1 MILS drastically reduces the quality of the view on laryngoscopy, impeding intubation in difficult airways. A bougie should be used routinely to minimise unnecessary manipulation of the C-spine.

2 RCCs have been shown to increase intracranial pressure by up to 4 mmHg by restricting venous outflow from the head. Depending on local policy, RCCs should be removed or loosened in patients with severe head injury, and head blocks and tape used alone. This situation is particularly important in patients who have been anaesthetised in the pre-hospital setting and are being ventilated.

3 RCCs may be detrimental in those with spinal deformities and the elderly (both groups have kyphosis, for example). Padding should be used to splint the neck in the position found.

4 Vomiting and aspiration is a serious risk of immobilisation. The RCC must usually be removed, and suction used, together with a head down or lateral tilt of the board with MILS applied.

5 There is some evidence to suggest that RCCs may restrict breathing, contribute to dysphagia, cause skin ulceration and pain, but these events are rare.

13 Basic airway management

Figure 13.1 Basic airway adjuncts

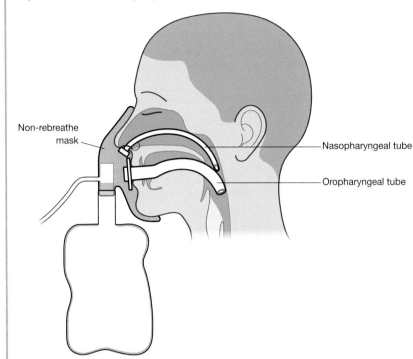

Non-rebreathe mask

Nasopharyngeal tube

Oropharyngeal tube

Upper airway obstruction

- Foreign body aspiration
- Blunt/penetrating laryngotracheal trauma
- Tonsillar hypertrophy
- Paralysis of vocal cords/folds
- Acute laryngotracheitis/bacterial tracheitis
- Epiglottitis
- Peritonsillar abscess
- Pertussis

Lower airway obstruction

- Foreign body aspiration
- Chronic bronchitis
- Bronchiectasis
- Asthma
- Bronchiolitis

Figure 13.2 Laryngeal mask airway (SAD)

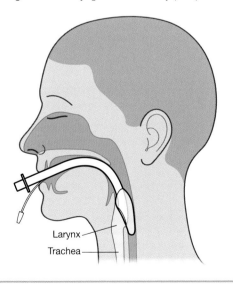

Larynx

Trachea

Figure 13.3 Endotracheal tube

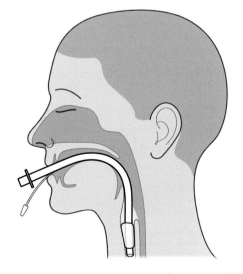

Pre-hospital Emergency Medicine at a Glance, First Edition. William Seligman, Sameer Ganatra, Timothy Parker and Syed Masud.
© 2018 John Wiley & Sons, Ltd. Published 2018 by John Wiley & Sons, Ltd.

Maintaining an oxygen supply to the heart, brain and other vital organs is of primary importance in critical care. Preserving a patent airway is thus paramount. In this chapter, we will consider how to identify a compromised airway and then work through the airway ladder, from manual airway manoeuvres to the use of airway devices. Discussion of the complex airway and failed airway drills is covered in other chapters.

Assessing the airway

When approaching the casualty, check for a response: a conscious, speaking patient is able to maintain his airway and needs no further airway manipulation. However, a patient's consciousness level may deteriorate rapidly at any time and regular reassessment of the airway is vital. If obtunded, the patient requires rapid airway assessment and management; a low GCS may be the cause or the result of a blocked airway.

Look, listen and feel when assessing the airway:

1. *Look* for: signs of neck or maxillofacial trauma; any obvious airway obstruction in the mouth (tongue, vomit, foreign body, tissue swelling); signs of increased respiratory effort (use of accessory muscles, tracheal tug, seesaw chest, intercostal and subclavian recession) which may be indicative of an airway (or breathing) problem.
2. *Listen* for: snoring (pharyngeal obstruction, typically by tongue); gurgling (fluid in airway); stridor (upper airway obstruction); absent breath sounds may also point to a blocked airway (or respiratory arrest).
3. *Feel* for: exhaled air on your cheek.

Manual airway opening manoeuvres

Pre-hospital management of the obstructed airway should begin with simple manoeuvres. *Head tilt and chin lift* improves airway alignment and moves the tongue away from the posterior pharyngeal wall respectively. With one hand gently placed on the forehead, the head is tilted back to the 'sniffing position', where the external auditory meatus is brought in line with the manubrium sterni. The chin is lifted vertically upwards between the thumb and two fingers: a common error here is to compress the soft tissues under the chin thereby occluding the airway. The chin lift should be avoided in trauma patients for fear of causing cervical spinal cord injury in those with suspected C-spine fractures.

The *jaw thrust* is an alternative manoeuvre to the chin lift suitable in those with suspected C-spine injuries. By placing four fingers behind the angle and ramus of the mandible, the jaw can be pushed anteriorly, while counter-pressure can be applied to the maxilla by the thenar eminences to prevent movement of the head. In this position it is easy to hold a face mask over the nose and mouth for oxygenation or ventilation.

In the absence of trauma, once the airway is open and if the patient is breathing, place them into the *recovery position*: this optimises airway patency by incorporating the chin lift and allowing gastric contents and secretions to leave the mouth rather than move down the trachea. If substantial fluid is present in the oropharynx, use a *Yankauer suction catheter* connected to a power source for drainage. Always suction under direct vision and for no longer than 15 seconds at a time in any patient to prevent tissue damage.

Basic airway adjuncts

Once the airway has been opened, adjuncts may be used to keep it open:

1 *Oropharyngeal (Guedel) airways (OPAs)* are designed to perform the role of a chin lift, keeping the tongue positioned forward. A correctly sized OPA should extend either from the corner of the patient's mouth to the tragus, or the centre of the incisors to the angle of the mandible. Insert one upside down and then rotate it by 180 degrees once in the mouth. Patients with an intact gag reflex will not tolerate OPAs; those who do are very likely to require prompt endotracheal intubation to provide definitive airway patency.
2 *Nasopharyngeal airways (NPAs)* are a useful adjunct in those patients for whom an OPA is unsuitable, i.e. those with intact gag reflexes. However, they are contraindicated in patients with suspected basal skull fractures. Look for Battle's sign, raccoon eyes, cerebrospinal fluid rhinorrhoea, new-onset cranial nerve deficits and other signs suggestive of a basal skull fracture before inserting an NPA. The device should first be lubricated and then inserted through the nostril, twisting it slightly to ease passage. An appropriately sized NPA should glide smoothly through the nostril without causing sustained bleeding.

Supraglottic airway devices (see Figure 13.1)

Supraglottic airway devices (SADs) are cuffed tubes that sit above the glottis. They comprise of laryngeal mask airways and I-Gels®. SADs present a trade-off: on the one hand, SADs allow for ventilation over the glottis and are ready to be inserted blindly without a laryngoscope and anaesthetic drugs; on the other, their cuffs do not protect the *lower* airways from aspiration of stomach contents, secretions or blood. This risk can be mitigated slightly by passing a nasogastric tube through the SAD, and intubation can take place with the device *in situ*, so that a SAD can be inserted while the intubation kit is being prepared.

Endotracheal intubation

Insertion of an endotracheal tube establishes a definitive airway, i.e. a cuffed tube in the trachea conferring patency and protection. Unlike the other airway devices, intubation requires extensive training, experience and regular practice, and must be performed only by pre-hospital care physicians and advanced care paramedics. Those with intubation skills must also be trained to manage the complications of intubation. The key is to not act beyond your own level of competence. The indications, procedure and complications of endotracheal intubation are discussed in detail in Chapter 26 on rapid sequence induction and pre-hospital anaesthesia.

14 The difficult airway

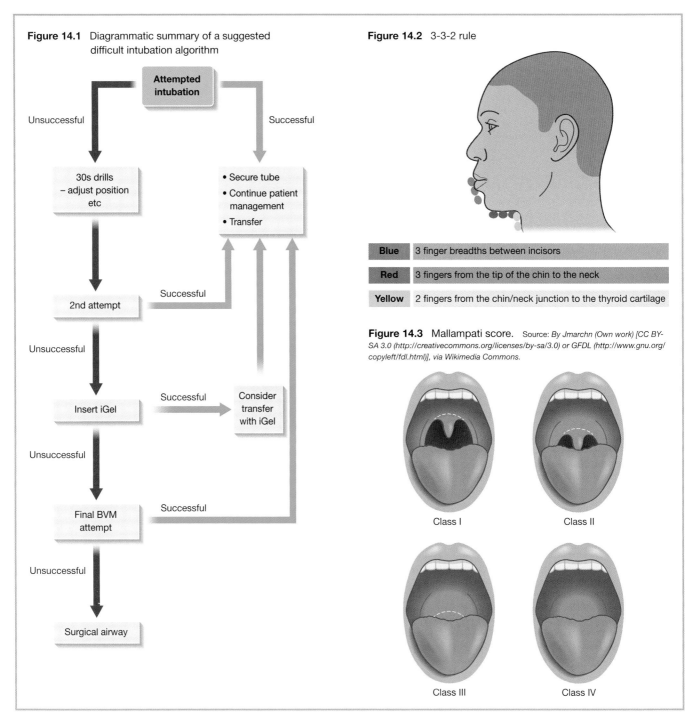

Figure 14.1 Diagrammatic summary of a suggested difficult intubation algorithm

- Attempted intubation
  - Unsuccessful
  - Successful
- 30s drills – adjust position etc
- Secure tube
- Continue patient management
- Transfer
- 2nd attempt
  - Successful
  - Unsuccessful
- Insert iGel
  - Successful
  - Unsuccessful
- Consider transfer with iGel
- Final BVM attempt
  - Successful
  - Unsuccessful
- Surgical airway

Figure 14.2 3-3-2 rule

Blue	3 finger breadths between incisors
Red	3 fingers from the tip of the chin to the neck
Yellow	2 fingers from the chin/neck junction to the thyroid cartilage

Figure 14.3 Mallampati score. Source: By Jmarchn (Own work) [CC BY-SA 3.0 (http://creativecommons.org/licenses/by-sa/3.0) or GFDL (http://www.gnu.org/copyleft/fdl.html)], via Wikimedia Commons.

Class I

Class II

Class III

Class IV

Pre-hospital Emergency Medicine at a Glance, First Edition. William Seligman, Sameer Ganatra, Timothy Parker and Syed Masud.
© 2018 John Wiley & Sons, Ltd. Published 2018 by John Wiley & Sons, Ltd.

Loss of an airway is a common cause of death for pre-hospital patients. *Airway management* is therefore a priority for pre-hospital care providers and, as previously explained, this can be achieved in a number of ways, ranging from simple manoeuvres, to the use of adjuncts and intubation. There are various definitions of a difficult airway, but for the purposes of this topic it is where a competent trained practitioner has difficulty with facemask ventilation, supraglottic airway device (SAD) ventilation, tracheal intubation, or all three. This is based on the American Society of Anaesthesiologists definition. Other definitions include "requiring more than 3 attempts to intubate" or "requiring more than 10 minutes to intubate". Pre-hospital practitioners must be able to predict and manage both expected and unexpected difficult airways. The following is a very brief overview as no algorithm or explanation can account for all the possible complex factors involved in a difficult airway.

Assessing the airway

Before selecting an airway management strategy, pre-hospital practitioners must assess how difficult they anticipate bag-valve-mask (BVM) ventilation, laryngoscopy, supraglottic device placement and cricothyroidotomy to be in a particular patient.

The following mnemonic (MOANS) helps to predict those patients in whom BVM ventilation may be difficult.

M – Mask seal difficulty, i.e. blood, facial injuries and facial hair
O – Obesity and Obstruction: obese and pregnant patients are more difficult to ventilate due to excess tissue/oedema
A – Age > 55: elderly patients are more difficult to ventilate due to decreased upper airway compliance
N – No teeth
S – Stiff lungs or stiff chest wall, snoring

The following mnemonic, LEMON (or LEMONS according to Berry) helps to predict those patients/scenarios in whom difficult laryngoscopy and intubation may be expected.

L – Look for obesity, receding jaw, short muscular neck, burns, facial trauma or macroglossia
E – Evaluate the 3-3-2 rule (Figure 14.2) to estimate the size of the oral cavity
M – Mallampati score (Figure 14.3) may not be particularly useful in the pre-hospital setting as it is assessed in a conscious, seated patient
O – Obstruction with blood, vomitus, oedema, a mass or foreign bodies
N – Neck mobility – may be restricted. With appropriate manual C-spine stabilisation, it is acceptable to undo a cervical collar during intubation
S – Space (confined or restricted), scene (location and lighting) and skill of the operator

Other mnemonics for predicting difficulty inserting supraglottic devices and surgical airway exist.

Difficult airway management

There are several different approaches to the management of a patient with a difficult airway described, including the UK Difficult Airway Society (DAS) Guidelines and the Vortex Approach among others (Figure 14.1). The level of management attempted will depend on the capability and training of the operator. In the first instance, the main effort should be directed to maintaining oxygenation of the patient.

The three main 'non-surgical' methods for maintaining an airway are:

1 Face-mask and bag-valve arrangement (usually self-inflating bag) +/– adjuncts/2 handed technique.
2 Supraglottic Airway Device (SAD), such as iGel® or laryngeal mask airway.
3 Endotracheal tube (ETT).

If a practitioner has taken the view that RSI is indicated, and the first attempt at intubation has failed, or a view of the cords has not been obtained, the following factors must be optimised. These are called the '30 second drills' as they must be completed in less than 30 seconds to reduce the likelihood of desaturation:

- adjust operator position/change operator
- adjust patient position
- use suction to clear contamination
- use stylet in place of bougie (see Chapter 26 on RSI)
- insert blade to maximum and slowly withdraw under vision
- external laryngeal manipulation (e.g. backward upward rightward pressure [BURP])
- release cricoid pressure
- long blade/McCoy blade/alternate laryngoscope, e.g. Airtraq™.

If these do not make subsequent intubation attempts successful, and the best attempts at oxygenation and ventilation with all three non-surgical methods fail after optimisation, or if the physiology, injuries and circumstances dictate, a surgical airway in the form of emergency cricothyroidotomy is usually indicated.

In some situations a SAD, e.g. iGel may be sufficient, or if a patient can be ventilated easily using BVM ventilation and the equipment is available, it may also be appropriate to attempt guided video-assisted intubation.

'Front of neck airway'

This should ideally only be attempted in the presence of full neuromuscular block or in critically injured patients near to death. The recommended technique in adults is scalpel cricothyroidotomy. Where the cricoid membrane is palpable, this may be done using a technique described by the DAS as 'stab, twist, bougie, tube', using a horizontal incision over the cricothyroid membrane. Where the cricoid membrane is not palpable, the technique becomes 'scalpel, finger, bougie, tube', using an elongated vertical incision to allow anatomical structures to be identified, prior to incision into the cricothyroid membrane. A detailed description of the technique is beyond the scope of this chapter.

An alternative technique, with limited application in the prehospital environment, is to use "needle cricothyroidotomy", where a suitably sized cannula is inserted into the trachea through the cricothyroid membrane. This will provide short term oxygenation only, and CO_2 levels will rise. In children under 12 this would be the preferred technique.

These techniques require appropriate training and rehearsal in a supervised setting.

15 Life-threatening chest trauma

Figure 15.1 The 6 immediately life-threatening types of chest injury (ATOMFC). Source: *see reference section.*

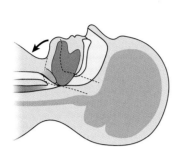

Airway obstruction

Loss of oropharyngeal tone is the most common cause of airway obstruction

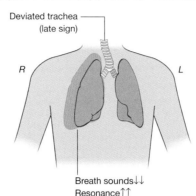

Deviated trachea (late sign)

Breath sounds↓↓
Resonance↑↑

Tension pneumothorax

Formation of a flap-valve causes air to enter the pleural space without a means of escape

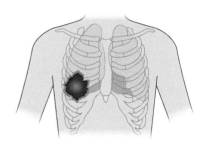

Requires 3 sided occlusive dressing

Open pneumothorax

Air follows the path of least resistance into the pleural cavity through large chest defects which remain open

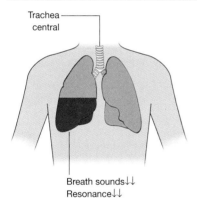

Trachea central

Breath sounds↓↓
Resonance↓↓

Massive haemothorax

Defined as >1.5 L initial chest drain output or >200 mLs/hr for 2–4 hours. Significant bleeding into the pleural space can compromise ventilation

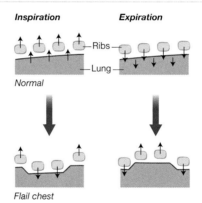

Inspiration   *Expiration*

Ribs
Lung
Normal

Flail chest

Flail chest

Fracture of >2 ribs each in >2 places results in a flail segment and paradoxical movement of the affected chest wall segment with breathing

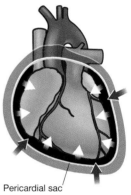

Shocked, muffled heart sounds, distended neck veins

Pericardial sac

Cardiac tamponade

Rapid accumulation of blood in the pericardial space via a ventricular defect prevents diastolic filling of the heart

Table 15.1 Potentially life-threatening chest injuries

Injury	Significance
Simple pneumothorax	May progress to tension
Traumatic aortic disruption	Risk of exsanguination, requires surgical/endovascular repair
Diaphragmatic rupture	Herniated abdominal organs may compress lungs/increase work of breathing
Tracheobronchial injury	Ongoing source of air leak may require multiple chest drains for lung decompression; risk of mediastinitis
Myocardial contusion	Decreased cardiac output
Pulmonary contusion	May cause progressively increasing ventilatory pressures

These further 6 injuries are potentially life-threatening and should be sought in the secondary survey. They are typically diagnosed and addressed in the hospital setting.

Pre-hospital Emergency Medicine at a Glance, First Edition. William Seligman, Sameer Ganatra, Timothy Parker and Syed Masud.
© 2018 John Wiley & Sons, Ltd. Published 2018 by John Wiley & Sons, Ltd.

Thoracic injury is a contributing factor in over half of all patients dying from trauma, with RTCs accounting for over 80% of all chest trauma sustained. Mortality in isolated chest trauma is in the region of 4–8%; however, the high energy impacts associated with thoracic injury in RTCs often affect additional multiple organ systems, in which case mortality increases to 35%.

Early recognition of chest injury is therefore of paramount importance in management of the trauma patient. However, patients in the pre-hospital phase rarely demonstrate the classic textbook signs associated with each of the specific pathologies, as injuries are seen in the early phase and are hence still evolving. Further, in the noisy pre-hospital environment, examination findings such as resonance and air entry are often too subtle for detection. A high index of suspicion must be applied to patients with potential chest trauma, aided by knowledge of kinematics and mechanisms of chest injury. An awareness of the importance of reading the scene in predicting injuries is thus crucial.

General principles of management

There are 12 distinct life-threatening thoracic injuries, known collectively as the 'deadly dozen'; six are immediately life-threatening, and six potentially life-threatening. In each case, general principles of management are directed at:

1 Maximising oxygen delivery, i.e. high flow oxygen and early intubation.
2 Avoiding ventilatory causes of cellular hypoxia, i.e. intubation and ventilation as necessary; if spontaneously ventilating, give adequate analgesia and ensure that there is no damage to the C-spine so that the patient can sit up and recruit lung bases for improved ventilation.
3 Alleviating any obstructive element of shock.

Immediately life-threatening chest trauma

Conventional wisdom dictates that there are six immediately life-threatening, but reversible, types of chest injury. These are often remembered using the mnemonic ATOMFC.

Airway obstruction

One in eight UK trauma patients have either partial or complete airway compromise at the point of admission to hospital. The most common cause of acute airway obstruction is impaired consciousness with loss of oropharyngeal tone and obstruction by the tongue. The priority is therefore to secure the airway rapidly using simple manoeuvres, adjuncts, or a definitive airway as indicated. Other causes of obstruction may include dentures, teeth, secretions, vomit or blood, which should be carefully removed/suctioned. Maxillofacial trauma, laryngeal trauma, airway oedema or expanding neck haematoma with airway compression will likely require a definitive airway.

Tension pneumothorax

Pathology: tension pneumothorax (TPx) occurs when a one-way-valve air leak occurs into the pleural space, either from the lung or through the chest wall. Air accumulates in the pleural space and exerts pressure on the ipsilateral lung, causing compression and mediastinal shift towards the contralateral side. This results in kinking of the great vessels and impaired venous return to the heart, with eventual circulatory collapse.
Causes: penetrating chest trauma, blunt chest trauma with parenchymal injury, iatrogenic (lung puncture, barotrauma from mechanical ventilation).

Signs: the classical triad of tracheal deviation, hyper-resonance and neck vein distension are late signs and are rarely seen. More commonly, the clinical course is one of chest pain, respiratory distress, rapid desaturation with tachycardia, reduced cardiac output and increasing ventilatory pressures. Focal chest signs and hypotension represent acute decompensation and rapidly precede circulatory collapse. Ventilated patients are observed to deteriorate faster than spontaneously breathing patients due to positive pressures.
Management: immediate needle decompression followed by tube (non-ventilated patients) or finger (ventilated patients) thoracostomy.

Open (sucking) chest wound

Pathology: a large open defect in the chest wall, measuring more than one-third of the diameter of the trachea, enables preferential entrainment of air via the wound into the pleural space. Air accumulates in the hemithorax, and intra- and extrathoracic pressures equilibrate, causing lung collapse.
Causes: penetrating chest trauma with large diameter open tract.
Signs: bubbling chest wound, profound hypoventilation and hypoxia, usually proportionate to the size of the defect.
Management: three-sided occlusive dressing to create a leaflet seal and tube thoracostomy.

Massive haemothorax

Pathology: large volume bleed into pleural space with compression of ipsilateral lung.
Causes: typically penetrating trauma.
Signs: shock, unilateral absence of breath sounds and dullness to percussion, flat neck veins.
Management: tube thoracostomy after resuscitation and blood transfusion. Secure good access as the thoracic cavity may hide very large volumes of blood with the possibility of rapid circulatory collapse on tube insertion. The tube should never be clamped to tamponade bleeding.

Flail chest

Pathology: multiple rib fractures (two or more ribs fractured in two or more places) resulting in loss of continuity of a segment of the chest wall with the thoracic cage. Hypoxia is caused by: voluntary splinting; associated pulmonary contusion; mechanically impaired chest wall movement.
Causes: typically high energy blunt trauma, e.g. frontal impact RTC, therefore often associated with underlying pulmonary contusion.
Signs: paradoxical movement of chest segment on inspiration, expiration and coughing. Also monitor for pneumo- and haemothorax.
Management: adequate analgesia and intubation/ventilation if profound ventilatory failure.

Cardiac tamponade

Pathology: bleeding into pericardial space, resulting in poor diastolic filling of the heart.
Causes: penetrating thoracic/upper abdominal injury.
Signs: traditional signs (Beck's triad of muffled heart sounds, distended neck veins and hypotension) are of limited value in the pre-hospital patient due to environmental noise. Witnessed loss of cardiac output following penetrating thoracic/upper abdominal injury makes the diagnosis likely.
Management: resuscitative clamshell thoracotomy.

16 Circulation I: haemodynamic instability

Figure 16.1 The pre-hospital blood box

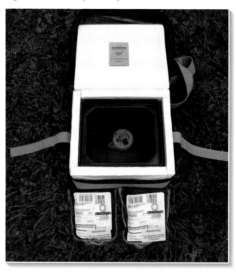

Table 16.1 Advantages and disadvantages of different fluids

	Advantages	Disadvantages
Crystalloid	Match plasma osmolality	Large volumes of normal saline lead to metabolic acidosis
Blood	If a patient is actively bleeding, replacing with blood is intuitive	Short shelf life Need for maintenance at precise temperature makes the use of pre-hospital blood logistically complex
Colloid	Contain large molecules which help retain fluid within intravascular space	Large molecules leak out of damaged capillaries causing resistant pulmonary and cerebral oedema
Dextrose	Helpful in resuscitating hypoglycaemic patients	Very little fluid stays in the intravascular compartment

Figure 16.2 Clotting cascade

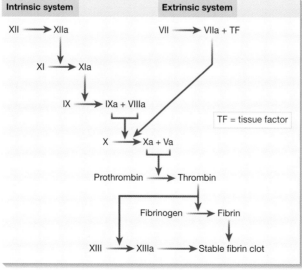

Source: Sander GE, Giles TD. Ximelagatran: Light at the End of the Tunnel or the Next Tunnel? *Am J Geriatr Cardiol*. 2004;13(4).

Pre-hospital Emergency Medicine at a Glance, First Edition. William Seligman, Sameer Ganatra, Timothy Parker and Syed Masud.
© 2018 John Wiley & Sons, Ltd. Published 2018 by John Wiley & Sons, Ltd.

Modern understanding of fluid resuscitation in trauma has developed largely from recent military conflicts. Early fluid resuscitation of haemodynamically compromised patients is of benefit. However, the volume and speed of fluid resuscitation is, as yet, not well defined.

Shock

Shock is defined as hypoperfusion of vital organs, i.e. not meeting the metabolic demands of vital organs including the heart and the brain.

Traditionally, pre-hospital care teams have relied on bedside measures of tissue perfusion to diagnose shock, e.g. blood pressure and heart rate. However, the best indicators of shock are plasma pH, end-tidal PCO_2, lactate and base excess. With point-of-care testing and capnography in pre-hospital care, it may now be possible for the pre-hospital team to access these vital pieces of information on the scene. This will allow more accurate assessment of the state of shock of a patient.

Suggested pre-hospital markers of shock

- pH – decreased (towards a further acidotic state)
- end-tidal PCO_2 – increased (as cardiac output decreases, elimination of CO_2 from the lungs decreases)
- lactate – increased with tissue hypoperfusion
- base excess – negative, i.e. base deficit due to by-products of anaerobic metabolism.

Types of shock

The body pumps a limited amount of blood around a series of closed loops. Shock may occur when blood is lost, the pump fails or the blood is distributed to the wrong loops.

Hypovolaemic shock

This is the most common type of shock seen in major trauma, often due to major haemorrhage. It may also occur in severe dehydration.

Cardiogenic shock

Pump failure may occur as a consequence of inflow obstruction (cardiac tamponade, tension pneumothorax), myocardial damage (myocardial infarction, heart failure) or outflow obstruction (pulmonary embolus, aortic dissection). The former type is sometimes classified as its own type of shock – obstructive shock.

Distributive shock

Blood may be distributed to the wrong tissues in a number of different clinical contexts. These include septic shock, spinal shock and anaphylaxis. In each of these situations, blood is diverted away from vital organs.

Permissive hypotension

Uncontrolled pressure changes will worsen haemorrhage. This is mainly due to the disruptive effect of high-pressure flow on established clots. Definitive haemostatic control may only be achieved in the operating theatre or radiology suite. Until that time, blood pressure should be kept at a level where cerebral and vital organ perfusion continues without harming clot formation. However, 'hypotensive resuscitation' should be balanced and not performed aggressively. This is particularly important with traumatic head injury patients in whom the benefits of adequate cerebral perfusion outweigh the benefits of aggressive 'hypotensive resuscitation'. When splinting and haemorrhage control have been optimised, intravenous fluids may be administered. Transfused blood is the fluid replacement of choice. However, if this is not possible then crystalloid should be used (Figure 16.1).

Haemostatic resuscitation

It is now established that the early use of blood and blood products as primary resuscitation fluids is beneficial. Early studies of Israeli trauma victims (Hirshberg *et al.* 2003) concluded that trauma patients with systolic blood pressure of 70 mmHg had already lost more than two-thirds of their blood volume. The use of blood as a resuscitation fluid is therefore intuitive. Several air ambulances now carry blood on board and it is typically given if each of the following criteria are met:

- systolic blood pressure < 90 mmHg at any time
- non-responder to fluid bolus
- suspected or confirmed haemorrhage.

Hirshberg's study suggests that pre-hospital blood transfusion is associated with improved outcome.

This study also suggested that preventing the profound coagulopathy of trauma (see Chapter 11, *Control of major haemorrhage*) required infusion of plasma before the patient became coagulopathic. There have been numerous subsequent studies that have shown the benefit of administration of fresh frozen plasma (FFP) with red blood cells in a ratio of 1:1. In the past, patients were likely to receive proportionately more red blood cells than FFP thereby diluting clotting factors, resulting in coagulopathy.

It has also been proven that use of tranexamic acid in major haemorrhage, if given in the first three hours after injury, is of significant benefit in reducing mortality in trauma patients. Tranexamic acid is now carried on all ambulances and administered routinely for haemorrhagic trauma. As a synthetic derivative of lysine, tranexamic acid blocks lysine binding sites on plasminogen preventing activation to plasmin (Figure 16.2).

Plasmin works to degrade fibrin, a protein that forms the framework of blood clots, and by preventing fibrin breakdown, tranexamic acid helps to support the clotting process.

17 Circulation II: medical cardiac arrest

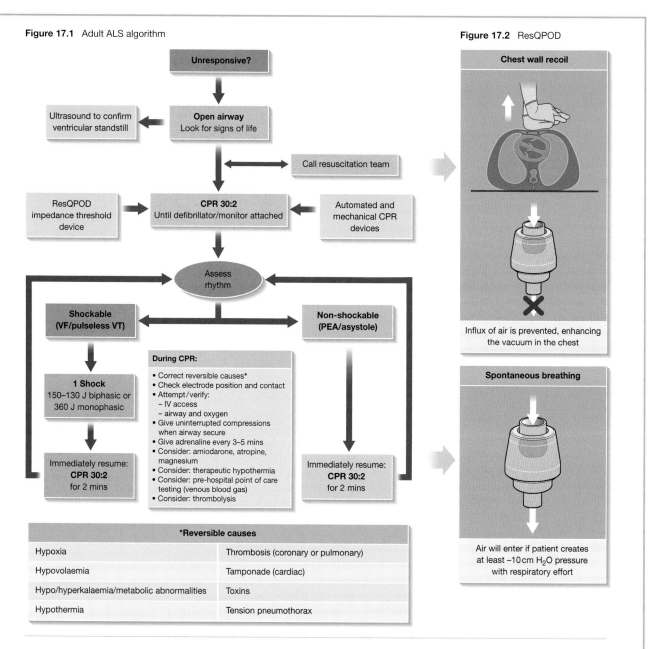

Figure 17.1 Adult ALS algorithm

```
                        Unresponsive?
                            │
                            ▼
Ultrasound to confirm  ◄── Open airway
ventricular standstill      Look for signs of life
                            │
                            ◄──────►  Call resuscitation team
                            │
ResQPOD                     ▼                    Automated and
impedance threshold  ───►  CPR 30:2        ◄───  mechanical CPR
device                     Until defibrillator/monitor attached   devices
                            │
                            ▼
                        Assess
                        rhythm
                    ┌──────┴──────┐
                    ▼             ▼
         Shockable              Non-shockable
         (VF/pulseless VT)      (PEA/asystole)
              │                      │
              ▼                      │
         1 Shock                     │
         150–130 J biphasic or       │
         360 J monophasic            │
              │                      │
              ▼                      ▼
         Immediately resume:    Immediately resume:
         CPR 30:2               CPR 30:2
         for 2 mins             for 2 mins
```

During CPR:
- Correct reversible causes*
- Check electrode position and contact
- Attempt/verify:
  – IV access
  – airway and oxygen
- Give uninterrupted compressions when airway secure
- Give adrenaline every 3–5 mins
- Consider: amiodarone, atropine, magnesium
- Consider: therapeutic hypothermia
- Consider: pre-hospital point of care testing (venous blood gas)
- Consider: thrombolysis

*Reversible causes	
Hypoxia	Thrombosis (coronary or pulmonary)
Hypovolaemia	Tamponade (cardiac)
Hypo/hyperkalaemia/metabolic abnormalities	Toxins
Hypothermia	Tension pneumothorax

Figure 17.2 ResQPOD

Chest wall recoil

Influx of air is prevented, enhancing the vacuum in the chest

Spontaneous breathing

Air will enter if patient creates at least −10 cm H_2O pressure with respiratory effort

Figure 17.3 Vscan

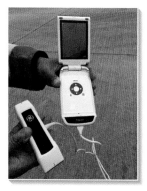

Figure 17.4 SonoSite

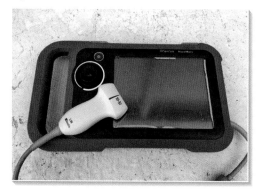

Pre-hospital Emergency Medicine at a Glance, First Edition. William Seligman, Sameer Ganatra, Timothy Parker and Syed Masud.
© 2018 John Wiley & Sons, Ltd. Published 2018 by John Wiley & Sons, Ltd.

Despite recent advances in our understanding of resuscitation, survival from out-of-hospital cardiac arrest still remains low. Centres in the UK that have used pre-hospital enhanced care teams to provide a primary cardiac arrest response have shown significant improvements in survival rates. However, currently there are not enough enhanced care teams to meet the demand from cardiac arrest cases in the UK. Several recent advances in resuscitation medicine are being used by enhanced care teams to improve survival from cardiac arrest.

Beyond advanced life support – enhanced cardiac arrest care

The vast majority of out-of-hospital cardiac arrests are managed by ambulance crews for whom the Resuscitation Council's advanced life support (ALS) algorithm dictates the care provided. However, enhanced care teams are able to supplement ALS protocols with several key interventions (Figure 17.1) which may improve survival and contribute to overall improved management.

Ultrasound

Technological advances have now made it possible for pocket ultrasound imaging to be utilised in the pre-hospital environment. Several studies have examined the use of ultrasound during cardiac arrest to detect potentially reversible causes. Although none of these studies has shown a survival benefit, if used at the right time by appropriately trained personnel, it can identify reversible causes of cardiac arrest. Indeed, the Resuscitation Council advocates the use of ultrasound when appropriately trained clinicians are available. However, ultrasound imaging should not interrupt or delay cardiopulmonary resuscitation (CPR). Placement of a subxiphoid probe just before chest compressions are paused for a planned rhythm check enables skilled operators to obtain vital views within seconds.

Automated cardiopulmonary resuscitation devices

Effective CPR is required to perfuse the heart and brain, to re-establish cardiac output and to achieve survival. Evidence suggests manual CPR by trained professionals achieves 25–30% of normal coronary and cerebral blood flow. Effective CPR during conveyance to hospital is very difficult to sustain. Automated devices may now be used to improve the quality of CPR. They can minimise the time without chest compression, provide a means of delivering more effective compressions during transport to hospital and allow the emergency services team to direct their efforts towards treating potentially reversible causes.

Inspiratory impedance threshold devices

Conventional CPR is inherently inefficient because just as the chest wall begins to recoil, air rushes in through an open airway and removes the negative pressure that is critical for returning blood to the heart. Impedance threshold devices limit air entry into the lungs during chest recoil between compressions (Figure 17.2). This decreases intrathoracic pressure and increases venous return to the heart.

Point of care testing

Some pre-hospital systems have capitalised on advances in the point-of-care blood testing industry to take the laboratory to the scene. Practitioners are able to analyse a patient's arterial blood to aid informed choice of ventilator settings, correct acid–base disturbances and in some cases measure cardiac enzymes (e.g. troponin) that are elevated in some myocardial infarctions.

Therapeutic hypothermia

There is some evidence that the use of induced mild hypothermia (32–34 °C for 12–24 hours) to treat hypoxaemic–ischaemic encephalopathy in comatose survivors of out-of-hospital ventricular fibrillation arrest is associated with improved neurological recovery. Cooling has also been shown to be of benefit when administered during cardiac arrest. Cooling can be achieved by the administration of ice-cold intravenous fluids in addition to the placement of ice packs. Invasive temperature monitoring should be undertaken using an oesophageal probe. It is necessary to sedate and paralyse patients who are cooled in order to prevent shivering which would otherwise cause re-warming.

Thrombolysis

Thrombolysis should be considered where the cause of cardiac arrest is thought to be a significant pulmonary embolus. Successful thrombolysis has been associated with improved neurological outcome. Thrombolytic drugs may take up to 90 minutes to take effect and therefore should only be administered if it is appropriate to continue CPR for this duration.

Post-return of spontaneous circulation care

Post cardiac-arrest syndrome describes the spectrum of organ dysfunction following return of spontaneous circulation (ROSC) in patients suffering a cardiac arrest. This includes brain injury, myocardial dysfunction, systemic ischaemic–reperfusion response and the persistence of any precipitating pathology. Interventions which address these components will improve survival and neurological outcome. Such interventions may include:

- airway protection and mechanical ventilation
- controlled reoxygenation (targeting saturations of 94–98%)
- targeted temperature management
- control of seizures
- control of blood glucose.

Although the prognosis for out-of-hospital cardiac arrest remains poor, the enhanced care capabilities delivered by specialist teams give patients the greatest chance of a better outcome. With the availability of point-of-care testing, ultrasound and devices that improve CPR, it is increasingly recognised that, where possible, cardiac arrests should be attended by enhanced care units utilising the paramedic–physician partnership.

18 Circulation III: traumatic cardiac arrest

Figure 18.1 Traumatic cardiac arrest algorithm

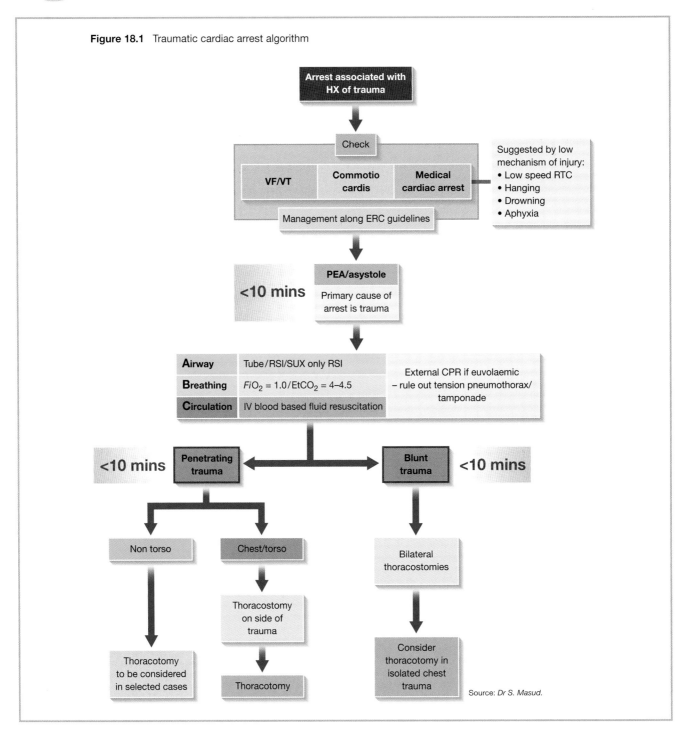

Pre-hospital Emergency Medicine at a Glance, First Edition. William Seligman, Sameer Tranatra, Timothy Parker and Syed Masud.
© 2018 John Wiley & Sons, Ltd. Published 2018 by John Wiley & Sons, Ltd.

Traumatic cardiac arrest – a different disease process to medical cardiac arrest

Until recently, many EMS systems have viewed attempting CPR in traumatic cardiac arrest (TCA) as a futile act given its high mortality. However, more recent research has shown that TCA has similar survival rates to medical cardiac arrest (Lockey *et al.* 2006).

An arrest associated with significant trauma may lead EMS to believe that it is a primary traumatic arrest. However, it is important to remember that a medical arrest may have precipitated the trauma. This must be considered particularly if the mechanism of injury is of low energy. For instance, a small RTC involving an elderly patient slumped over the steering wheel may have been the result of a myocardial infarction.

Until recently, TCA was considered as following the same disease process as medical cardiac arrest and was managed similarly. However, TCA is an unique disease that occurs as a result of damage to a previously healthy heart. This differs from medical cardiac arrests, the most common cause for which is pre-existing ischaemic coronary artery disease. In TCA, the healthy heart may have arrested as a result of hypoxia, haemorrhage or obstructive shock. If these causes are dealt with promptly, the greater the chance that a previously healthy heart will start functioning again. The commonest causes of medical and TCAs are listed and compared in Table 18.1.

The priority in managing a patient in whom one suspects primary TCA is to reverse the cause of the arrest as listed in Table 18.1. An algorithm (Figure 18.1) that fits the causes of TCA should be followed just as strictly as would be expected of ALS providers in in-hospital medical arrests. However, the content of the algorithm should be adjusted in order to prioritise the primary causes of TCA.

Recognition of cardiac arrest

The use of pre-hospital ultrasound is greatly enhancing our ability to diagnose peri-arrest and cardiac arrest states. While it may sometimes be difficult in the pre-hospital environment to determine whether a patient has a pulse or not, an effectively trained operator can diagnose cardiac standstill rapidly and unequivocally at the scene using basic ultrasound.

Key principles in the management of traumatic cardiac arrest

The procedures that must be carried out, without exception, in the pre-hospital setting are oxygenation and fluid resuscitation. Control of these factors may involve more advanced procedures such as intubation (RSI), thoracostomy and thoracotomy. CPR is not the priority in TCA. This is because in the context of the causes of traumatic arrests, the presence of hypovolaemia, tension pneumothorax or pericardial tamponade will all limit venous return, left ventricular end-diastolic volume and therefore the effectiveness of chest compressions. External chest compressions may also delay definitive interventions, e.g. thoracotomy and, in the presence of chest trauma, may even exacerbate underlying injuries and pathology.

However, just as with medical cardiac arrests, the response expected by responders varies significantly with their level of training and experience. While basic life support providers will provide CPR and rescue breaths, ALS providers will consider intubation and the use of drugs. Currently, only enhanced care units will deliver the advanced care that TCAs require. Enhanced care units will be composed of a doctor trained in PHEM as well as an advanced paramedic. First responders will not do any harm by following basic life support. However, given that the interventions suggested are all time-critical and potentially life saving, the aim should be to deliver the appropriately trained team with the necessary qualifications and experience to provide this gold-standard enhanced care in the pre-hospital environment. Timely and appropriate focused interventions will ensure the best chance for victims of TCA to survive.

Return of spontaneous circulation and on-going management and transfer

Should these resuscitative measures be successful and the return of spontaneous circulation be achieved, the subsequent immediate management and transfer of the patient to hospital are equally important. Continued advanced airway and ventilation support will be imperative. Patients will need to be anaesthetised, further volume resuscitated if required, and normothermia maintained before transfer to the appropriate hospital can begin. The decision over whether to transport the patient to hospital by helicopter (if available) or road ambulance is governed by both clinical factors, e.g. whether stability has been achieved or whether further invasive interventions are likely to be required, and environmental factors, e.g. the location of the incident, the weather and the resources available. Ultimately, critically ill patients who may require interventions during transfer to hospital will be best transported by land ambulance.

Table 18.1 Commonest causes of medical and TCAs

Medical cardiac arrest	Traumatic cardiac arrest
Coronary artery disease	Hypoxia
Arrhythmia – primary or secondary	Hypovolaemia (exsanguination/ hypovolaemic shock)
Valvular heart disease	Tension pneumothorax
Cardiomyopathy	Pericardial tamponade

19 Pain relief and sedation

Figure 19.1 WHO pain ladder with prehospital adjustments. Source: *Cancer pain relief. WHO (1986). Reproduced with permission of WHO.*

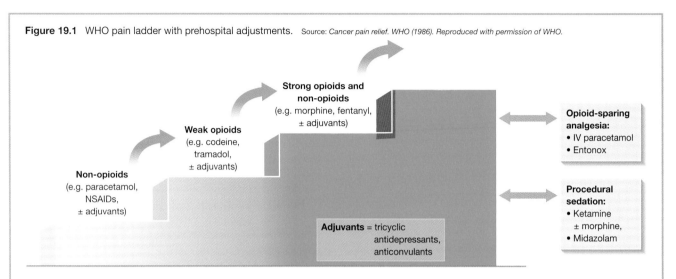

Table 19.1 Commonly used analgesics in pre-hospital care (including sedatives)

Drug	Mechanism	Dose	Contraindications	Key side effects	Toxicity
Paracetamol	COX inhibitor	1 g QDS PO/IV	No major contraindications	Rare	Hepatotoxicity in overdose
Entonox	Unknown	Self-titrated (INH)	Enclosed air spaces: pneumothorax, intracranial air (head injury), decompression sickness	Drowsiness, nausea; inhibition of B12, folate, and DNA synthesis (long-term use only)	Rare
Fentanyl	μ agonist	1–2 μg/kg IV	Respiratory depression	Nausea, constipation, drowsiness, miosis	Respiratory depression, hypotension
Morphine	μ agonist, GABA antagonist, and more	2.5–5 mg IV; titrate to pain	As for fentanyl	As for fentanyl	As for fentanyl
Ketamine	Non-competitive NMDA antagonist	0.25–5 mg/kg IV/IO	Hypertension, severe cardiac disease, stroke; raised intracranial pressure; head trauma; acute porphyria	Tachycardia, hypertension, hypersalivation (affecting airway management), increased muscle tone (affecting extrication), emergence phenomena	Respiratory depression, CNS effects (mild agitation to coma)
Midazolam	GABA agonist	1–2 mg IV/IO	Severe respiratory depression or disease	Drowsiness, confusion	Respiratory depression

Box 19.1 Assessing pain

- Pain must be assessed and reassessed ideally every 5 minutes during care, paying particular attention to the trend in pain scores.
- Age-appropriate assessment tools should be used to score pain: in adults and older children, self-report scales such as the numeric rating scale or visual analogue scale should be used, whilst Wong-Baker Faces may be used for younger children.
- The key is to communicate regularly with the patient: if this is not possible (e.g. unconscious patients), do not assume that the patient is not in pain, and prescribe appropriate analgesia for the degree of injury predicted.

Figure 19.2 Pain scale. Source: *Whaley and Wong's* Nursing Care of Infants and Children. Reproduced with permission of Elsevier.

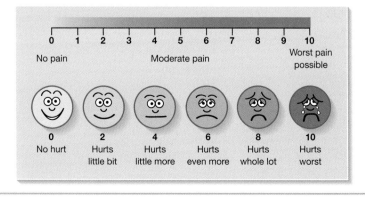

Pre-hospital Emergency Medicine at a Glance, First Edition. William Seligman, Sameer Ganatra, Timothy Parker and Syed Masud.
© 2018 John Wiley & Sons, Ltd. Published 2018 by John Wiley & Sons, Ltd.

Pain is often managed suboptimally in the pre-hospital environment. This is most commonly due to the pre-hospital care practitioner underestimating the patient's condition, opting for inadequate pain relief, or for fear of overdosing on analgesia. It is now well documented that effective pain control improves patient outcomes and that pre-hospital care practitioners require a firm understanding of how to assess and manage pain.

Importance of pain relief

It is a natural instinct for medical professionals to want to alleviate a patient's pain. However, there are further advantages to pain relief:

1 *Psychological*: further painful interventions and handling will not be received well by a patient already in pain. Timely pain management may also reduce cases of post-traumatic stress disorder and other chronic pain states.

2 *Physiological*: the sensation of pain triggers an 'injury response', wherein catecholamines and steroids are released and the immune system is activated to prepare the body to deal with stress. While beneficial in the short term, excessive stimulation by unrelieved pain can worsen patient outcome. Prolonged sympathoactivation can result in myocardial ischaemia and worsen head injury. Analgesia may also improve outcomes directly, for example in chest wall injuries, where pain relief may facilitate ventilation and adequate oxygenation.

3 *Practical*: a patient who is not distressed will help all involved to administer treatment calmly and effectively.

Non-pharmacological pain relief

Simple non-pharmacological measures can complement analgesics, reducing the dosages required and potentially minimising side-effects. Reassurance and empathetic communication can alleviate distress and can distract the patient from their discomfort. The reassuring presence of a parent can work in a similar way for paediatric casualties.

Pharmacological analgesia

Healthcare professionals usually turn to the WHO's analgesic ladder (Figure 19.1) for guidance when managing pain relief. However, in the acute, pre-hospital setting, other considerations such as speed of onset and ease of administration in the field come to the fore, and so the ladder appears quite different.

Paracetamol and non-steroidal inflammatory drugs (NSAIDs) are not used as commonly in the pre-hospital environment as in hospital due to their relatively slow onset. Intravenous paracetamol may be used as an opioid-sparing agent.

Entonox is a 50:50 mixture of oxygen and nitrous oxide and is an inhalational analgesic. With a rapid onset and offset, it is often used while preparing means of longer-lasting pain relief or to provide short-term supplementary analgesia during difficult handling or interventions. It is easy to titrate and patients can self-administer it. As Entonox is used exclusively in the short-term in the pre-hospital environment, side-effects are minimal; however, if therapeutic exposure to Entonox exceeds 24 hours, or if the analgesic is used more frequently than every four days, vitamin synthesis, particularly B12 and folate, can be inhibited and bone marrow function impaired.

Opiates like morphine and fentanyl are commonly administered. Morphine is considered the original opiate analgesic, but fentanyl is often preferred in the field. It has an almost immediate onset of action when given intravenously and lasts for up to an hour. Patients given fentanyl should be transferred to hospital accompanied by the administrating practitioner.

Ketamine is a dissociative anaesthetic which has a rapid onset of action (one minute) and a short duration (15–30 minutes), making it the ideal analgesic for short periods of intense pain (e.g. extrication, chest drain insertion). It can also be used for procedural sedation. With a large therapeutic index, ketamine toxicity is rare in the clinical setting. Key side-effects include hypertension, tachycardia, hypersalivation and increased muscle tone, as well as emergence phenomena such as vivid dreams, hallucinations and dysphoria. Due to its potent analgesic and psychoactive properties, ketamine is often used in combination with morphine and midazolam: morphine complements the dissociative effects of ketamine while enhancing the total pain relief administered; midazolam eases the unpleasant psychoactive side-effects.

Local anaesthetics have a very limited role in prehospital analgesia. They may be used topically before inserting cannulae in children and needle-phobic adults, as well as in peripheral nerve blocks. These allow for profound pain relief of a local area without the need for sedation. However, a combination of effective splintage and strong opiates and ketamine is usually quicker and easier to administer.

Procedural sedation

Sedation is used to relieve agitation which might otherwise impede particular procedures, e.g. chest drain insertion. It is also used specifically after intubation to suppress a sympathetic response, reduce cerebral oxygen requirement, and prevent recall of the distressing events. Patients are usually moderately sedated in the pre-hospital environment such that there is no compromise to airway, breathing, or circulation. All patients undergoing sedation will require monitoring of non-invasive blood pressure or at least presence of radial pulse, ECG, pulse oximetry and end-tidal carbon dioxide, as well as regular verbal and visual (respiratory rate, alertness, responsiveness to pain) contact. Practitioners should also be vigilant for signs of inadequate sedation: hypertension, tachycardia, mydriasis, lacrimation and perspiration. The equipment used for RSI and resuscitation should be available. Critically, only those trained in RSI and tracheal intubation should be allowed to carry out procedural sedation in the unstable, isolated pre-hospital setting. A range of drugs used in varying combinations may be used to sedate a patient, but there are a few common principles:

• medications must be administered intravenously wherever possible as this is the most efficient route

• doses should be titrated to effect

• all syringes must be labelled with the name of the drug and its concentration.

20 Head injury

Figure 20.1 Reading the scene

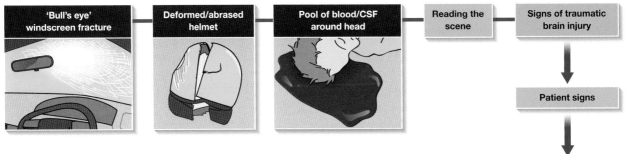

| 'Bull's eye' windscreen fracture | Deformed/abrased helmet | Pool of blood/CSF around head |

Reading the scene → Signs of traumatic brain injury → Patient signs

Table 20.1 Glasgow Coma Scale. Source: *Adapted from http://www.glasgowcomascale.org/*

Behaviour	Response	Score
Eye opening	Spontaneous	4
	To speech	3
	To pain	2
	No response	1
Best response: verbal	Fully oriented	5
	Confused speech	4
	Inappropriate words	3
	Incomprehensible sounds	2
	No response	1
Best response: motor	Obeys commands	6
	Localises to painful stimulus	5
	Withdraws from painful stimulus	4
	Flexes to pain (decorticate)	3
	Extends to pain (decerebrate)	2
	No response	1
Severity of TBI	Minor brain injury	13–15
	Moderate brain injury	9–12
	Severe brain injury	3–8

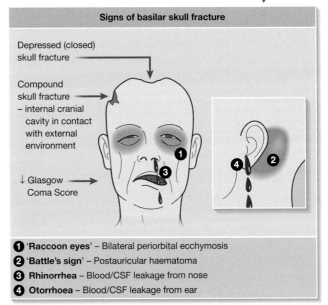

Signs of basilar skull fracture

Depressed (closed) skull fracture

Compound skull fracture – internal cranial cavity in contact with external environment

↓ Glasgow Coma Score

1 **'Raccoon eyes'** – Bilateral periorbital ecchymosis
2 **'Battle's sign'** – Postauricular haematoma
3 **Rhinorrhea** – Blood/CSF leakage from nose
4 **Otorrhoea** – Blood/CSF leakage from ear

Figure 20.2 Classification of primary traumatic brain injury. Sources: *see reference section.*

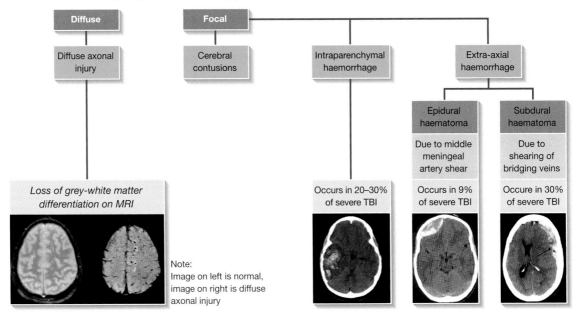

Diffuse → Diffuse axonal injury → *Loss of grey-white matter differentiation on MRI*

Note: Image on left is normal, image on right is diffuse axonal injury

Focal → Cerebral contusions | Intraparenchymal haemorrhage (Occurs in 20–30% of severe TBI) | Extra-axial haemorrhage

Epidural haematoma – Due to middle meningeal artery shear – Occurs in 9% of severe TBI

Subdural haematoma – Due to shearing of bridging veins – Occure in 30% of severe TBI

Pre-hospital Emergency Medicine at a Glance, First Edition. William Seligman, Sameer Ganatra, Timothy Parker and Syed Masud.
© 2018 John Wiley & Sons, Ltd. Published 2018 by John Wiley & Sons, Ltd.

Fifty percent of all patients dying from major trauma die as a direct result of significant head injury. Mortality in severe traumatic brain injury (TBI), defined as a GCS <8, approaches 50%. Optimal management in the pre-hospital phase is absolutely paramount in minimising the high burden of mortality and morbidity associated with head injury.

Demographics and aetiology

Traumatic brain injuries occur mainly in men (70–88%), who are 3.4 times more likely to die than women from these injuries. Alcohol is involved in up to 65% of all cases of TBI. Other causes include road traffic collisions, falls and assaults. These statistics are helpful in predicting those patients at risk of sustaining head injury even before arriving on the scene, where equating mechanism of injury with injury prediction will allow effective treatment and intervention. The likelihood and severity of TBI is indicated by the important clues from reading the scene before the patient is assessed for specific symptoms and signs of head injury.

Primary vs secondary brain injury

Primary brain injury

Primary brain injury refers to the physical damage at the initial point of insult. This may be either from blunt or penetrating trauma with damage occurring directly at the site of impact, or indirectly, from movement of the brain within the skull, resulting in cerebral contusions (coup-contrecoup). Shearing and rotational forces as the head is rapidly accelerated and decelerated cause disruption of blood vessels and axons, causing intracranial haemorrhage (ICH) and diffuse axonal injury. Primary brain injury can only be prevented by public health education initiatives, e.g. wearing cycle helmets, etc.

Secondary brain injury

This is the damage caused by the physiological and anatomical changes occurring at any time after the initial injury. These include: hypoxia; hypotension; raised intracranial pressure (ICP, due to ICH/cerebral oedema); and excitotoxicity (seizures). Secondary brain injury is potentially reversible and must be treated in order to minimise mortality and morbidity from the initial insult.

Assessment

The GCS provides an objective measure of a patient's conscious level. Repeat assessment of the head-injured patient's GCS is essential in determining both immediate management and prognosis. A GCS <8 is typically associated with a loss of protective airway reflexes requiring intubation, while the initial motor score holds the greatest prognostic value. Frequent reassessment is pivotal in the pre-hospital phase as patients may deteriorate rapidly. An initial GCS of 14 may be reassuring, but one in five such patients have ICH confirmed on later computed tomography (CT). Therefore, based on prediction of likely clinical course, patients assessed as at risk of serious TBI will be anaesthetised by enhanced care teams despite a reasonably high GCS on initial arrival at the scene. This is especially of significance in the agitated and combative patient, with early consideration of the likely clinical course critical in determining the immediate management, i.e. requirement to intubate early.

Pupils should be regularly assessed for signs of raised ICP. A unilaterally sluggish/fixed, dilated pupil (or indeed any other evolving focal neurology) is indicative of rising ICP and most likely evolving ICH and must be managed urgently.

Management priorities

After the primary insult, hypoxia and hypotension are the leading causes of mortality in TBI. These are exacerbated by raised ICP, and as such, management is directed at careful optimisation of these parameters.

1 *Airway protection and oxygenation*: GCS <8 requires RSI and intubation (consider carefully); target saturations 100% (lower saturations are correlated with increasing mortality); C-spine immobilisation. All patients sustaining any trauma above the base of the neck must be assumed to have a C-spine injury until otherwise proven.
2 *Ventilation*: meticulous control of low–normal CO_2 (3.5–4.0 kPa) to control ICP – this is achieved by control of respiratory rate, tidal volumes and inspiratory:expiratory ratios.
3 *Correction of hypovolaemia and hypotension*: careful fluid administration to maintain systolic blood pressure of 100 mmHg (single episode of hypotension <90 systolic doubles mortality).
4 *Reduce ICP*: loosen C-spine collar to reduce venous congestion; transport at 45 degrees; consider use of hypertonic saline in cases of evolving focal neurology; controversially, early pre-hospital burr hole surgery to reduce ICP has been proposed by some in very particular circumstances, e.g. long transfer time/distance to trauma centre.
5 *Early transfer to neurosurgical centre*: ideally, CT of the head within 1 hour followed by immediate appropriate neurosurgical intervention as directed by scan.

Additional considerations

Agitated head injuries: agitated head injury patients are at significant risk of acute deterioration requiring urgent neurosurgical intervention. In such a state, these patients cannot be transported to hospital by helicopter as there is both insufficient space to allow advanced airway management once the patient is loaded, and a danger to the aircraft and its crew. Combative patients may further put themselves at risk through a lack of effective C-spine immobilisation and even greater increase in ICP. As such, it is often a difficult clinical judgement as to whether to sedate the patient, e.g. with morphine and midazolam, with a view to RSI and intubation to effect rapid transfer to hospital via helicopter, or to transport the patient by land such that there is scope to secure the airway in the back of the ambulance in the event of deterioration.

Maxillofacial trauma: head injuries are often accompanied by significant maxillofacial trauma. Face and scalp lacerations can result in substantial blood loss due to the tense fascia around the head keeping bleeding vessels open. Excessive nasopharyngeal haemorrhage may obstruct the airway and obscure views despite suction, and may require packing with inflatable balloon devices. Hard palate fractures should be manually reduced to control haemorrhage and splinted with bite blocks.

21 Spinal injuries

Figure 21.1 Diagram of dermatomes. Source: *Faiz O, Blackburn S, Moffat D.* Anatomy at a Glance, 3rd edition *(2011). Reproduced with permission of John Wiley & Sons.*

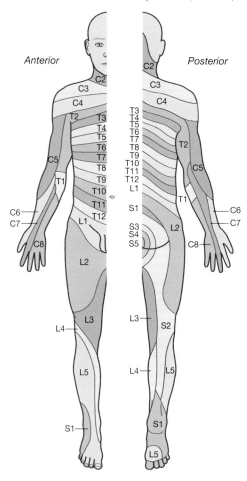

Table 21.1 Primary cord syndromes

Syndrome	Arterial insufficiency	Mechanism of injury	Sensory deficit	Notes
Anterior cord syndrome	Anterior spinal artery	Hyperflexion/rotation: compression from fracture of vertebral body or anterior dislocation of intervertebral disc	Complete motor paralysis, reduced pain and temperature	Typically seen in roll-over or motorcycle accidents, or falls from horses. Worst prognosis of the four cord syndromes: only 10–15% of patients demonstrate any functional recovery
Posterior cord syndrome	Posterior spinal artery	Hyperextension: posterior vertebral body fractures	Proprioception and fine touch (with resulting sensory ataxia)	Rare
Central cord syndrome		Hyperextension: usually in elderly with osteoarthritic spine (cervical spondylosis)	Motor (flaccid paralysis), pain and temperature	Central cord is pinched between osteophytes from the vertebral body and the thick ligamentum flavum. Due to the relatively central position of cervical tracts, the upper limbs are affected more than the lower limbs
Brown-Séquard syndrome		Penetrating injuries and lateral mass fractures: hemisection of cord	Ipsilateral motor, fine touch, and proprioception, contralateral pain and temperature	

Pre-hospital Emergency Medicine at a Glance, First Edition. William Seligman, Sameer Ganatra, Timothy Parker and Syed Masud.
© 2018 John Wiley & Sons, Ltd. Published 2018 by John Wiley & Sons, Ltd.

Spinal cord injuries (SCI) can have a devastating impact on long-term mobility and independence. The most commonly affected group are young males between 16 and 30 years old, as they are most likely to be the victims of trauma. Road traffic collisions account for half of all SCI. However, the ageing population means that rising numbers of active elderly people are becoming involved in trauma and are particularly vulnerable to SCI. This is because of comorbidities such as osteoporosis, osteoarthritis of the spine and cervical spondylosis. As a result, SCI are a growing problem with an increasingly diverse demographic picture.

Anatomy of the spine and cord

The spinal column functions to support the upper body as well as to protect the spinal cord. There are 33 vertebrae which surround the cord: 12 thoracic, 7 cervical, 5 lumbar, 5 sacral, and 4 coccygeal (fused) vertebrae. These are supported by intervertebral discs and ligaments. The cord itself runs within the spinal canal from the foramen magnum at the base of the brainstem to the level of L1 in adults, below which the canal is occupied by the cauda equina. The spinal cord is made up of various tracts, some afferent, others efferent, which branch off to give sensory and motor innervation to specific dermatomes and myotomes, respectively. As well as sensory and motor nerves, the cord also contains autonomic nerve fibres: the sympathetic fibres originate between T1 and L3, and the parasympathetic between S2 and S4.

Pathophysiology of cord injury

There are four main mechanisms of blunt injury: hyperflexion, hyperextension, rotation and compression. These may be seen in high-speed road traffic collisions or sporting incidents. The cord is most likely to be damaged at the points of transition (cervicothoracic, thoracolumbar, lumbosacral junctions), for it is at these points that the prevailing mobility of the spine changes. For instance, rotation in the thoracic spine switches to flexion/extension in the lumbar spine.

Primary spinal cord injury

Primary SCI occurs at the time of impact, and can be due to either blunt or penetrating injury. The functional sequelae of primary SCI depends on the vertebral level of the lesion as well as the tracts that are affected. In terms of the latter, four key syndromes exist: anterior cord, posterior cord, central cord and Brown-Séquard syndromes (Box 21.1).

Secondary spinal cord injury

Secondary SCI is caused by further mechanical disruption, hypoxia and hypoperfusion of the cord after the initial injury. These three factors can extend the area of primary injury through causing oedema with resultant ischaemia of the cord.

SCI management in the pre-hospital phase and beyond is aimed at preventing secondary SCI.

Spinal shock

Spinal shock is a transient reflex depression of cord function. Within 24–72 hours of the primary injury, there is loss of anal tone, bladder and bowel function, and sustained priapism.

Neurogenic shock

Neurogenic shock refers to a triad of hypotension, bradycardia and hypothermia. This is due to vasodilation which results from loss of sympathetic outflow and unopposed vagal parasympathetic tone. This occurs in significant injuries at T6 or above.

Management of spinal cord injury

Management always begins with prompt neurological assessment: elicit the mechanism of injury and any pain or other neurological symptoms from the patient. Perform a formal examination of limb movements, sensory level and inspect for deformity. In the unconscious patient, look for evidence of neurogenic shock, diaphragmatic breathing, priapism (often partial), and flaccid paralysis with absent reflexes. The unconscious trauma patient should always be presumed to have sustained SCI. Wherever possible, the neurological assessment should be carried out prior to sedation or anaesthesia and documented thoroughly for legal purposes.

The treatment of SCI should be aimed at minimising secondary SCI. Spinal immobilisation measures are described in Chapter 12, and further equipment is shown opposite. Attention should also be paid to preventing further mechanical disruption to the spinal cord while the patient is in transit, and a balance should be struck between smooth driving and the arrival time at hospital. SCI should otherwise be managed using an ABCDE approach:

1 *Airway:* ensure airway is patent without unnecessary manipulation of the C-spine. Always use a bougie and be prepared to settle for a view of the arytenoids.
2 *Breathing:* spinal cord is neurological tissue and may suffer secondary hypoxic neurological damage in the same way as the brain. Titrate oxygen saturations to 100%. If the patient is complaining of being – or appears – short of breath, look for diaphragmatic breathing, as this may indicate a high cervical lesion (C3–C5). Have a low threshold for intubation in these patients, especially if there is concurrent chest trauma.
3 *Circulation:* hypotension (<100 mmHg) should be corrected by fluid resuscitation. If SCI is confirmed – and all other causes of hypotension excluded – inotropic support may be initiated.
4 *Disability:* check blood glucose and administer dextrose if patient is hypoglycaemic.
5 *Exposure:* consider that SCI patients will lose the ability to thermoregulate if autonomic function is impaired, and so should be kept warm. Expose the patient and carry out a full top-to-toe examination, but restrict the duration of full exposure to the minimum required in order to lessen the potential for hypothermia.

22 Limb injuries

Figure 22.1 Kendrick traction device

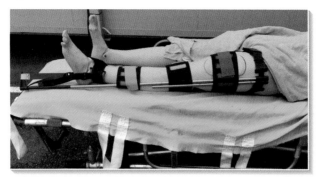

- Unilateral femoral shaft fractures (open or closed)
- Can be used in the presence of a confirmed or suspected pelvic fracture
- Contraindicated in presence of ankle fracture

Figure 22.2 Box splint

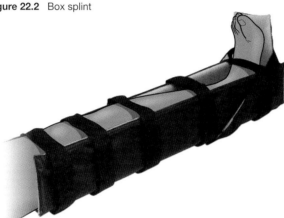

- Several sizes available according to locally agreed equipment lists
- Limb fractures with minimal displacement and instability
- Situations in which it is difficult or contraindicated to apply traction splinting
- If a more suitable splint is not available

Figure 22.3 Vacuum splint

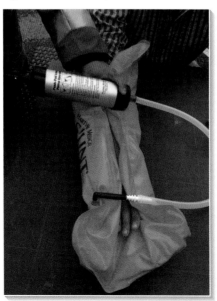

- Most limb fractures, particularly if displaced, angulated or unstable

Pre-hospital Emergency Medicine at a Glance, First Edition. William Seligman, Sameer Ganatra, Timothy Parker and Syed Masud.
© 2018 John Wiley & Sons, Ltd. Published 2018 by John Wiley & Sons, Ltd.

Limb injuries are commonplace and range from minor sprains to traumatic amputations. Pre-hospital care practitioners should be prepared to treat the entire range of limb injuries whilst maintaining appropriate overall clinical priority.

Primary survey

The ABCDE approach (see Chapter 21) should always be adopted as initial management. The exception to this is massive external haemorrhage where time spent performing assessment of airway and breathing would put the patient at risk of death from exsanguination. In this case, stop the haemorrhage first by progressing up the haemostatic ladder (see Chapter 11) and then transfer the patient urgently to the nearest trauma centre with an appropriate pre-alert message.

Secondary survey

Having addressed any life-threatening issues in the primary survey, the secondary survey should be carried out. Full exposure of the patient is important. This will allow for complete assessment of all four limbs for injury.

Wound care

Any abrasion or laceration may represent an open (compound) fracture. Any gross contamination should be washed away with normal saline. The wound should be dressed with sterile, saline-soaked, dressings. Tetanus injections are not given in the pre-hospital environment, and antibiotics may or may not be given depending on local pre-hospital protocols.

Fractures and dislocations

Limb deformity should be identifiable from rapid assessment, signifying long bone fractures or dislocations. Remove all jewellery from the injured limb before swelling occurs. The distal neurovascular status of the affected limb should be determined immediately and documented. If compromised, urgent realignment of the limb to the anatomical position ought to be performed after provision of adequate analgesia with or without sedation depending on the presence of enhanced care teams. The limb can be manipulated using longitudinal traction and manual correction. Distal neurovascular status must be rechecked after realignment and once again documented.

Analgesia

Before any manipulation of an injured limb, appropriate analgesia must be given. Options for analgesia can include Entonox, opiates and procedural sedation. Procedural sedation must be delivered by an enhanced care team led by a pre-hospital care physician. Drugs considered for sedation include ketamine and midazolam. During the procedure, appropriate monitoring must be attached.

Splintage and packaging

Bringing deformed limbs back into anatomical alignment prevents further haemorrhage and neural damage from the mobile ends of fractured bones damaging blood vessels and nerves, and also minimises the area into which any torn blood vessels can bleed. Immobilisation reduces pain by eliminating unnecessary movement at fracture sites. Splintage is a means of maintaining fractured limbs in the anatomical arrangement and preventing unstable fractures or dislocations from slipping back into their original positions. It also may be necessary in cases where the current position of the displaced limb or joint is impeding patient packaging and transport.

There is a variety of methods for splinting injured limbs. Upper limb injuries may be splinted most easily by the patient holding their limb in the most comfortable position; a triangular bandage can be used to support the limb. In forearm and lower limb fractures, specialised splints exist, each with different indications. The advantages and disadvantages of each are explained opposite.

Finally, the patient should be transferred to the hospital that best serves their clinical needs. For instance, a patient with an open fracture and significant soft tissue injury or an amputation should be treated at a centre with plastic and orthopaedic surgical expertise.

Other scenarios

Amputation

Amputations may be traumatic (partial or complete) or therapeutic. In all cases, the stump should be dressed and haemorrhage arrested. The amputated limb should be maintained in the best possible condition (free of gross contamination, double-bagged with ice in the second bag to ensure safe cooling) in order to allow reimplantation surgery with minimal tissue damage. Time-critical amputations may be carried out in the field where retaining the limb would be fatal. If time allows, it is recommended that two senior pre-hospital physicians make the decision to amputate. Deep sedation or general field anaesthesia is mandatory. The equipment required comprises of an arterial tourniquet, scalpel, Gigli bone saw, tuff cut scissors, and several pairs of haemostats. A surgical team from the nearest trauma hospital may be considered.

Crush injury

The severity of crush injury is proportional to the scale and duration of crush. Muscle damage leads to rhabdomyolysis, hyperkalaemia, myoglobinaemia and hypovolaemia. The majority of these effects will be delayed; effective management of crush injuries in the pre-hospital environment must prioritise intravenous fluid replacement.

Fat embolism

Fat embolism can occur following major long bone fractures, manifesting with pulmonary and cerebral compromise often with skin petechiae. Effective splintage and correction of hypoxia and hypovolaemia can correct this otherwise potentially fatal syndrome.

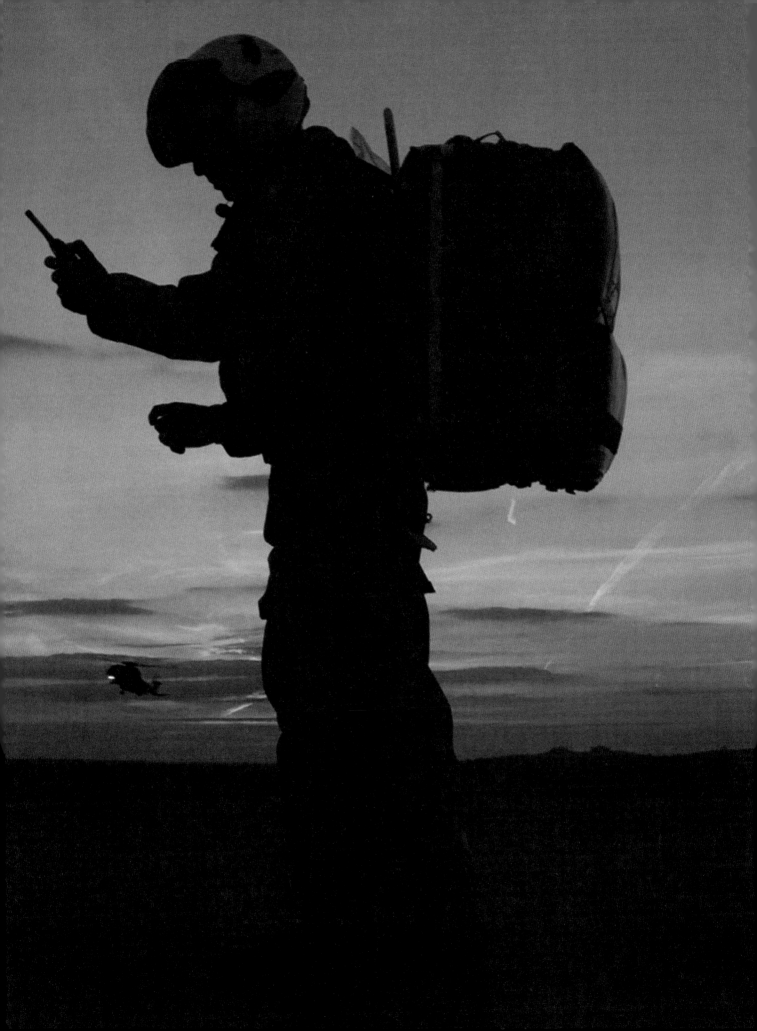

Special considerations in trauma management

Part 3

Chapters

23 Paediatric trauma

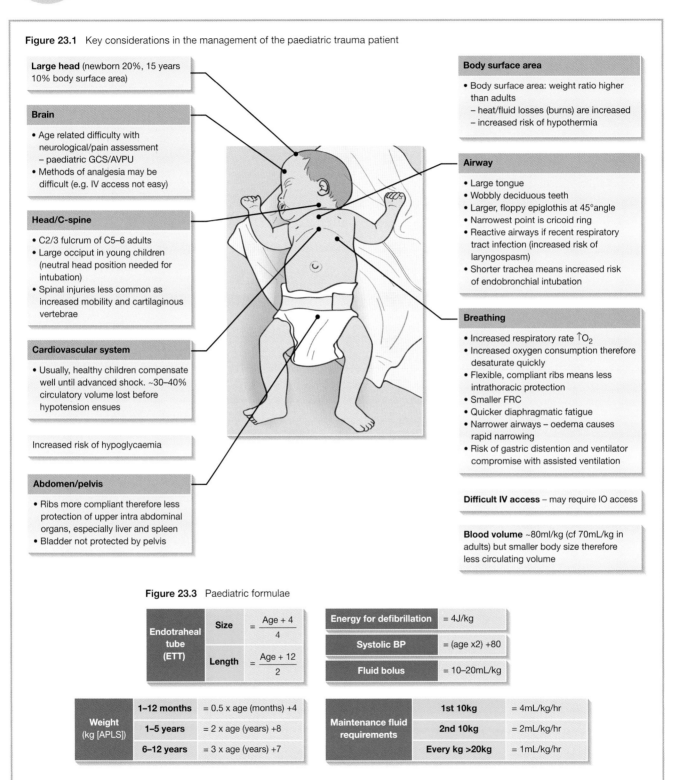

Figure 23.1 Key considerations in the management of the paediatric trauma patient

Large head (newborn 20%, 15 years 10% body surface area)

Brain

- Age related difficulty with neurological/pain assessment
  – paediatric GCS/AVPU
- Methods of analgesia may be difficult (e.g. IV access not easy)

Head/C-spine

- C2/3 fulcrum of C5–6 adults
- Large occiput in young children (neutral head position needed for intubation)
- Spinal injuries less common as increased mobility and cartilaginous vertebrae

Cardiovascular system

- Usually, healthy children compensate well until advanced shock. ~30–40% circulatory volume lost before hypotension ensues

Increased risk of hypoglycaemia

Abdomen/pelvis

- Ribs more compliant therefore less protection of upper intra abdominal organs, especially liver and spleen
- Bladder not protected by pelvis

Body surface area

- Body surface area: weight ratio higher than adults
  – heat/fluid losses (burns) are increased
  – increased risk of hypothermia

Airway

- Large tongue
- Wobbly deciduous teeth
- Larger, floppy epiglothis at 45°angle
- Narrowest point is cricoid ring
- Reactive airways if recent respiratory tract infection (increased risk of laryngospasm)
- Shorter trachea means increased risk of endobronchial intubation

Breathing

- Increased respiratory rate ↑O_2
- Increased oxygen consumption therefore desaturate quickly
- Flexible, compliant ribs means less intrathoracic protection
- Smaller FRC
- Quicker diaphragmatic fatigue
- Narrower airways – oedema causes rapid narrowing
- Risk of gastric distention and ventilator compromise with assisted ventilation

Difficult IV access – may require IO access

Blood volume ~80ml/kg (cf 70mL/kg in adults) but smaller body size therefore less circulating volume

Figure 23.3 Paediatric formulae

Endotraheal tube (ETT)	Size	$= \dfrac{Age + 4}{4}$
	Length	$= \dfrac{Age + 12}{2}$

Energy for defibrillation	= 4J/kg
Systolic BP	= (age x2) +80
Fluid bolus	= 10–20mL/kg

Weight (kg [APLS])	1–12 months	= 0.5 x age (months) +4
	1–5 years	= 2 x age (years) +8
	6–12 years	= 3 x age (years) +7

Maintenance fluid requirements	1st 10kg	= 4mL/kg/hr
	2nd 10kg	= 2mL/kg/hr
	Every kg >20kg	= 1mL/kg/hr

Pre-hospital Emergency Medicine at a Glance, First Edition. William Seligman, Sameer Ganatra, Timothy Parker and Syed Masud.
© 2018 John Wiley & Sons, Ltd. Published 2018 by John Wiley & Sons, Ltd.

The analogy that 'children are just small adults' is often used. However, when it comes to trauma management, there are anatomical, physiological and psychological differences that must be taken into account, although the basics remain very similar to adults. Emotional involvement can be very difficult to avoid as can bystander and parental pressure. Non-accidental injury and safeguarding issues may also be a feature. The wide range in size from a newborn to a 16 year old makes triage difficult.

Body size and weight

From a preterm infant weighing only a few kilos to an adult-sized teenager, paediatric body sizes and proportions vary vastly. Infants have a much larger head in relation to the size of their body (20%) and the relative contribution to overall body surface area decreases with age to adult proportions (10%) by adolescence. Children have a higher surface area to weight ratio than adults which means they are more susceptible to heat loss and hypothermia, in addition to fluid loss in burns. Various formulae (Figure 23.1) exist to aid estimation of weight, and equipment such as Broselow or Sandell tapes are available to assist.

Figure 23.2 Using a Broselow tape.
Source: By Stkittschris (Own work) [CC BY-SA 3.0 (http://creativecommons.org/licenses/by-sa/3.0)], via Wikimedia Commons.

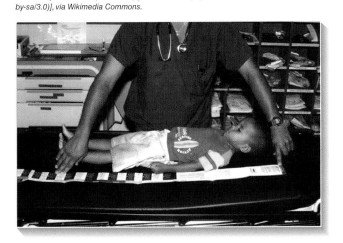

Airway

Children have an increased risk of airway obstruction due to large tongues, smaller mid face, smaller airway diameters, frequent respiratory tract infections and adenotonsillar hypertrophy. The larynx is higher and more anterior than adults and the narrowest point is the cricoid ring. The trachea is shorter and less rigid, making compression and endobronchial intubation more common. The large occiput in babies and young children may produce excessive flexion, causing tracheal compression and therefore neutral head positioning is used for intubation of young children. Deciduous teeth may be loose and the epiglottis is proportionately larger and more floppy.

Respiratory system

Ribs are more compliant and offer less protection to underlying organs. They are less likely to fracture than adults but there can be significant damage to underlying viscera without fracture. The smaller functional residual capacity and increased oxygen consumption make desaturation more rapid. Gastric distension can significantly compromise ventilation.

Cardiovascular system

Vital signs vary with age, making triage difficult (Figure 23.3). Young children have higher blood volumes per kilogram, but smaller circulating volumes overall.

Neurological system

Assessment of neurological status is difficult in babies and young children. The AVPU system or paediatric GCS can be used. Spinal injury is less common in children due to cartilaginous vertebral bodies, elastic ligaments and more mobility of the verbal column, distributing force over a wider area

Non-accidental injury

Unfortunately, paediatric trauma may be the result of NAI and responders should be alert to safeguarding issues. A careful history of how the injury occurred must be taken. Any concern that the trauma may have happened as a result of NAI should be documented and relayed to the receiving hospital team.

Paediatric primary survey

Airway

Children are more susceptible to airway obstruction and more rapid desaturation, therefore management of the airway should be performed swiftly if there is any sign of compromise. Rapid sequence intubation should only be performed by those confident in paediatric intubation within a pre-hospital setting due to the additional difficulties posed by the paediatric patient. Cuffed endotracheal tubes are safe in the short term and are more likely to be sized correctly in the first instance (Table 23.1) and they provide more airway protection where there is a risk of airway soiling or difficulties with ventilation. Care should be taken with assisted ventilation not to insufflate air into the stomach since gastric distension can splint the diaphragm and make ventilation more difficult. A nasogastric tube may be inserted after intubation to decompress the stomach.

Table 23.1 Laryngeal mask airway (LMA)

Weight (kg)	LMA size	Cuff volume (mL)
>5 kg	1	4
5–10	1.5	7
10–20	2	10
20–30	2.5	14
30–50	3	20

Breathing

Signs of respiratory distress in children include use of accessory muscles, tracheal tug, grunting and nasal flaring, intercostal muscle recession, and peripheral and central cyanosis. Paediatric BVMs should be used where available with a mask of an appropriate size and with caution to avoid over-distension and barotrauma.

Circulation

Hypotension may not develop until 25–40% of circulating volume has been lost. Peripheral perfusion is a useful sign of circulatory compromise. Intravenous access can be difficult in young children and may be made more difficult in hypovolaemia. Intraosseous access should be considered after two attempts or more than 90 seconds of attempting intravenous access. In hypovolaemia, a 20 mg/kg fluid bolus should be given. There is no evidence of benefit from smaller fluid boluses (in the same way practitioners permit hypotension in some bleeding adults) in paediatric practice.

Abdominal injuries are more likely as there is less protection for the upper abdominal organs from the compliant thoracic cage leading to an increased likelihood of splenic and liver injuries. The pelvis protects the bladder less effectively than in adults.

Disability

Head injuries are common in children but assessment of neurological status may be difficult in young children. An alternative GCS scoring system adapted specifically for children may be considered for greater accuracy. Hypoglycaemia is more common in children.

Burns

Assess the burn area using Lund and Browder charts which takes age into account. The rule of nines is inappropriate in young children given the larger head surface area. A child's palm and fingers is a useful estimation of 1% total body surface area. The higher surface area to weight ratio leads to increased fluid loss from burn areas. Smaller airway diameter means that airway obstruction occurs more quickly with inhalational burns and intubation should be performed promptly.

Spinal injury

The risk of high cervical spine fractures is high due to the larger head. Weak neck muscles mean that the fulcrum of spinal flexion is C2/3 in smaller children and C5/6 in older children. Great care should be taken to immobilise children at the pre-hospital stage. Spinal cord injuries are also possible without radiological abnormalities (SCIWORA). Car seats, adult lower limb box splints and vacuum splints are useful for the immobilisation of babies and toddlers.

Analgesia

Pain and distress should be ameliorated as quickly as possible. Use of Entonox may be considered in children old enough to be able to use it and intranasal diamorphine is a useful drug if intravenous access is difficult.

Consent and parents

Keeping parents close by is useful to reduce distress for the child and to enable consent and information gathering. Children under 16 who are deemed competent can consent to treatment (Gillick competence) but cannot refuse treatment. Emergency treatment should be provided where necessary, ideally with consent of the person with parental responsibility. However, they may not be present. Parental presence at resuscitation attempts may be beneficial and aid grieving when outcomes are unsuccessful.

Box 23.1 Emergency drug doses

Adrenaline (resuscitation dose) bolus 10 mcg/kg (0.1 mL/kg 1:10,000)
Amiodarone loading dose 5 mg/kg
Atracurium 0.5 mg/kg
Atropine 20 mcg/kg (minimum 100 mcg, maximum 600 mcg)
Bicarbonate (resuscitation dose) 1 mL/kg 8.4%
Calcium chloride 0.2 mL/kg 10% (slow IV)
Calcium gluconate 0.5 mL/kg 10% (slow IV)
Diazepam 0.1–0.25 mg/kg IV, 0.5 mg/kg rectally
Dextrose 2 mL/kg 10% IV
Ketamine* 2 mg/kg
Lorazepam 0.1 mg/kg (maximum 4 mg)
Magnesium 25–50 mg/kg (maximum 2 g)
Mannitol 250–500 mg/kg (1.25–2.5 mL/kg of 20%) over 30 mins
Midazolam 0.5 mg/kg (maximum 20 mg)
Naloxone 10 mcg/kg IV
Phenytoin (loading) 18 mg/kg IV over >30 mins
Prednisolone 1–2 mg/kg PO (maximum 40 mg)
Propofol* 2–4 mg/kg IV
Rocuronium 0.6 mg/kg IV
Salbutamol 2.5–5 mg nebulised, 5 mcg/kg bolus IV

*Doses of induction drugs are for guidance only should be administered with caution in patients with cardiac disease and haemodynamic instability.

24 Trauma in the pregnant woman

Figure 24.1 Key considerations in the management of trauma in the pregnant woman.

Source: *Holbery N and Newcombe P. Emergency Nursing at a Glance (2016). Reproduced with permission of John Wiley & Sons.*

Neurological

- Altered drug handling
- Decreased anaesthetic/analgesic drug requirements (20–40%)

Respiratory system

- Decreased FRC due to upward displacement of diaphragm by gravid uterus (~4cm)
- Diaphragmatic displacement – thoracostomies should be performed higher up
- Increased O_2 consumption + decreased FRC means faster desaturation
- Increased respiratory rate ~15%, increased tidal volume ~40% means reduced $PaCO_2$ (normal 4.1 kPa in pregnancy)

Haematological

- 40% increase in plasma volume – can lose ~1500ml before signs of hypovolaemia
- Dilutional physiological anaemia
- Increased risk of venothrombo-embolism (increased factors VIII, IX, X, fibrinogen and decreased antithrombin III and proteins)
- Decreased platelet count (dilution and consumption)
- Pregnancy induced coagulopathies (e.g. HELLP syndrome – haemolysis elevated liver enzymes and low platelets)

Foetus/uteroplacental unit

- CTG/foetal HR useful assessment of maternal circulatory status

Airway

- Increased risk of difficult and failed intubation (1:250)
- Large breasts – difficult laryngoscopy
- Oedamotous tissues of larynx
- Increased risk of epistaxis with nasal/airway adjuncts
- Increased risk of aspiration

Cardiovascular system

- Aortocaval compression when supine means decreased cardiac output due to decreased venous return
- 50% increase in cardiac output by 3rd trimester
- Decreased SVR (oestrogen/progesterone effect)
- 15–25% increased HR
- Stroke volume increase ~30–35%
- Cardiac apex moves to left – left axis deviation, ST depression and T wave inversion

Abdomen

- Increased intragastric pressure means increased risk of aspiration
- Risk of direct foetal injury, placental abruption and early labour
- Placental abruption may lead to mixing of foetal/maternal blood and requirement for Anti D if Rhesus negative
- Placental perfusion is dependent on maternal blood pressure and circulating volume (foetal heart rate is an early indicator of maternal hypovolaemia)
- Risk of concealed haemorrhage
- Abdominal examination is likely to be unreliable

Perimortem caesarean section

- Should be attempted in any pregnant woman >20 weeks or in practice any woman with a visible pregnancy as unlikely to be able to ascertain gestation
- <23 weeks increases maternal survival
- >23 weeks increased maternal and neonatal survival
- Should be started after 4 minutes loss of circulation
- Paediatric team will be needed for neonatal resuscitation

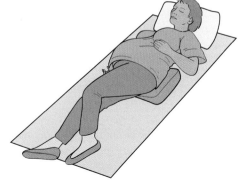
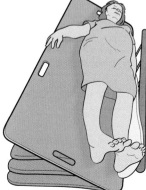

Trauma in a pregnant patient in the late second or third trimester should ideally be managed in a major trauma centre with an obstetric department, to allow further obstetric and neonatal management. The pre-alert from the pre-hospital care team must request that these specialists are part of the receiving trauma team. The physiological and anatomical changes of pregnancy impact on the management of trauma in a number of ways.

Physiological and anatomical changes in pregnancy relevant to trauma

Airway
Capillary engorgement of the mucosa of the pharynx and larynx leads to oedema and increased risk of bleeding (epistaxis can occur with the use of nasal airways). Increased breast size and oedematous airway mucosa lead to an increase in the frequency of difficult and failed intubations. Use of a stubby handled blade or removal of the blade of the laryngoscope from the handle and reattaching once the blade is in the oropharynx may help. In addition, there is an increased risk of aspiration due to raised intragastric pressure from the expanding uterus and hormone-related reduced oesophageal sphincter pressures. Desaturation occurs more rapidly due to the reduction in functional residual capacity and increased oxygen consumption by approximately 20% to 300 mL/minute at term.

Respiratory system
Functional residual capacity is reduced by the upwards displacement of the diaphragm by the uterus (approximately 4 cm). The respiratory rate is increased by approximately 15% at term and tidal volume increases by about 40% leading to a physiological respiratory alkalosis with a $PaCO_2$ of approximately 4 kPa in pregnancy. Thoracostomies should be performed at a higher level due to the upwards displacement of the diaphragm.

Cardiovascular system
Stroke volume increases by more than 30% due to increased circulating volume. Cardiac output is increased by approximately 50% at term and so the relative reserve for further stress on the myocardium is limited. Blood pressure falls secondary to progesterone-mediated vasodilatation and decreased systemic vascular resistance from the first trimester onwards, increasing back to normal levels by the third trimester. Vena cava compression by the uterus can reduce cardiac output in mid-trimester women by up to 30%. Because of this, pregnant trauma patients must be managed in the left lateral position to minimise compression and therefore hypotension (Figure 24.1).

The increase in circulating volume means that there is an increased ability to compensate for haemorrhage: systolic blood pressure may only fall after 30–40% of the circulating volume is lost (approximately 2000 mL) after which rapid decompensation results. Hypotension in a pregnant woman in the face of trauma should be treated aggressively, taking the increased circulating volume into account. Concealed haemorrhage may occur in abdominal trauma, e.g. placental abruption. The foetal blood supply is not autoregulated and is dependent on maternal mean arterial pressure, thus monitoring the cardiotocography and foetal heart rate are useful early indicators of maternal circulatory compromise. The cardiac apex is displaced to the left and anteriorly, resulting in left axis deviation and sometimes ST segment depression and T wave inversion on the ECG.

Haematological system
A dilutional physiological anaemia results from the greater increase in plasma volume (50%) compared with the increase in red cell mass (30%). Pregnancy and the puerperium are hypercoagulable states. There is a risk of disseminated intravascular coagulation due to thromboplastin and plasminogen activator release. Combined with trauma, the risk of thromboembolism is much increased and prophylaxis in the form of low molecular weight heparin, compression stockings and intermittent compression boots should be considered where mobilisation is likely to be delayed.

Abdomen and pelvis
The uterus rises out of the pelvis by approximately 12 weeks' gestation, when it becomes vulnerable to blunt abdominal trauma. The uterus and amniotic fluid can absorb some force; however, the placenta can shear resulting in placental abruption. Abruption may be heralded by uterine contractions, as bleeding is an irritant to uterine muscle. Bleeding may show per vagina or be concealed. Blunt trauma can also cause preterm labour, preterm rupture of membranes and increased risk of uterine rupture, especially if a uterine scar is present. The bladder is pushed upwards and is also more liable to injury. Pelvic fracture can result in bony fragments which can cause direct foetal injuries. The increase in circulating volume leads to splenic engorgement and increased risk of splenic injury and ensuing intraperitoneal haemorrhage. The foetus is also at increased risk in the case of maternal electrocution given the amniotic fluid sac within which it lies.

Trauma may cause foetal haemorrhage which can lead to foetal anaemia and potentially foetal exsanguination and death. Mixing of foetal and maternal blood can also occur and if the mother is Rhesus negative, she will require administration of anti-D immunoglobulin as soon as possible.

Neurological
There is a reduction in anaesthetic and analgesic requirements by approximately 20–49% during pregnancy. Therefore caution should be exercised with sedation doses of anaesthetic agents, as general anaesthesia may result.

Perimortem caesarean section
Loss of cardiac output in a pregnant woman of more than 20 weeks' gestation should prompt consideration of early resuscitative perimortem caesarean section. In practice this means any visibly pregnant woman, as the exact gestation is unlikely to be known. This procedure increases maternal survival only before 23 weeks' gestation; after this a survival benefit for the foetus is incurred. Ideally the procedure should be commenced within 4 minutes of loss of circulation and completed within 5 minutes. A paediatric resuscitation team will be needed for the neonate.

Neonatal life support (see Figure 24.2)

Figure 24.2 Newborn life support algorithm.
Source: *Resuscitation Council Reproduced with permission of the Resuscitation Council (UK).*

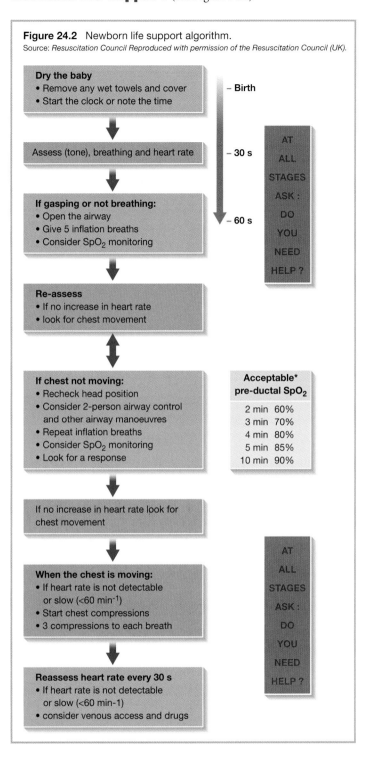

25 Trauma in the elderly

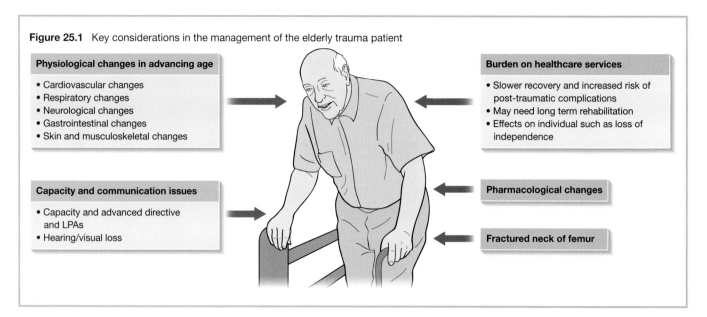

Figure 25.1 Key considerations in the management of the elderly trauma patient

Physiological changes in advancing age

- Cardiovascular changes
- Respiratory changes
- Neurological changes
- Gastrointestinal changes
- Skin and musculoskeletal changes

Burden on healthcare services

- Slower recovery and increased risk of post-traumatic complications
- May need long term rehabilitation
- Effects on individual such as loss of independence

Capacity and communication issues

- Capacity and advanced directive and LPAs
- Hearing/visual loss

Pharmacological changes

Fractured neck of femur

Relatively minor falls or seemingly unimportant incidents, often not recalled, may cause significant trauma in the elderly. Injuries may be missed or underestimated.

Physiological changes with advancing age

Ageing leads to progressive functional decline and reduced physiological reserve. Frailty is a risk factor for ongoing complications and slower recovery.

Cardiovascular changes

- Reduced compliance and impaired ventricular diastolic filling, lead to lower cardiac output reserve. Tachycardia exacerbates the decrease in cardiac output.
- Downregulation of beta-adrenoceptors leads to reduced response to inotropic drugs and a profound reduction in cardiac output on induction of anaesthesia.
- Higher resting diastolic and systolic blood pressures. Hypovolaemic shock may be relatively masked with hypotension representing a greater blood loss than in a normotensive individual.
- Arrhythmias are more common due to fibrosis of cardiac conducting tissue. Atrial fibrillation (AF) is common. Sympathetic stimulation increases the risk of arrhythmias and both lead to reduced cardiac output and compromised myocardial blood supply. Furthermore AF increases the risk of venous thromboembolism post-trauma.
- Pulse pressure is widened due to atherosclerosis of blood vessels. This can mask the narrowing of pulse pressure that results in hypovolaemic shock.
- Coronary blood flow is reduced due to degenerative calcification, thickening of the tunica intima and atherosclerosis. This means that in the face of hypotension, cardiac ischaemia is more likely than in healthy individuals.

- Desensitisation of baroreceptors in the carotid sinuses and aortic arch means that reflex responses to hypotension are reduced. Induction of anaesthesia, particularly in the face of hypotension, can induce profound hypotension.
- Normal responses to hypovolaemia may be masked by drugs: beta blockers may prevent tachycardia in response to hypovolaemia; antihypertensives may exacerbate hypotension.

Respiratory changes

- Structural changes in the airways with ageing lead to an increased tendency for airway collapse during sleep and anaesthesia. These changes also increase airway compliance, leading to compression of small airways and closure during expiration resulting in air trapping. The residual volume increases, as does the functional residual capacity (larger oxygen reservoir if full pre-oxygenation is possible).
- Respiratory muscles are weaker in the elderly.
- Volume of the pulmonary vasculature decreases and the pulmonary vascular resistance increases significantly (approximately 75%) as does pulmonary artery pressure (25%).
- Reduced alveolar surface area as a result of small airway dilatation leads to a worsening of gas exchange.
- FVC and FEV1 are reduced.
- Arterial PO_2 is reduced but PCO_2 remains the same.
- Difficult BVM ventilation can occur in edentulous patients and impaired neck mobility can lead to difficulties with intubation.

Neurological system

- Degeneration and atrophy of grey matter accompanied by an increase in cerebrospinal fluid (CSF) volume means the brain has relatively more space within the cranium. Head injury is more

Pre-hospital Emergency Medicine at a Glance, First Edition. William Seligman, Sameer Ganatra, Timothy Parker and Syed Masud.
© 2018 John Wiley & Sons, Ltd. Published 2018 by John Wiley & Sons, Ltd.

likely to lead to dural venous bleeding since vessels are more vulnerable to shearing forces.

- Cerebral blood flow is reduced, especially if cerebrovascular disease is present.
- Cerebral oxygen demand is reduced.
- Autoregulation is usually maintained.
- Reduced volume and structural change occur in the spinal cord. Spinal cord ischaemia during episodes of hypotension is more likely with co-existing cardiovascular changes of ageing.
- Pathology such as cervical spondylosis may be present leading to myelopathy and pre-existing neurological changes complicating neurological assessment.
- Memory loss, dementia and hearing or visual impairment may be present making communication difficult.
- Autonomic nervous system: reduced re-uptake of catecholamines and increased sympathetic basal activity combined with a progressive decline in the parasympathetic nervous system.

Renal system

- Reduced cortical blood flow means increased likelihood of acute renal failure as a result of prolonged or profound autoregulation.
- Fluid and electrolyte imbalance may exist due to medication such as diuretics, compounded by poor dietary intake and reduced thirst.
- With a background of relative potassium retention due to aldosterone deficiency secondary to reduced renin secretion, tissue damage and crush injuries can lead to dangerously elevated serum potassium levels.

Gastrointestinal system

- Reduced hepatic and splanchnic blood flow lead to increased likelihood of ischaemia when hypotensive episodes occur.
- Reduced albumin and alpha-1 acid glycoprotein concentrations lead to altered drug handling.
- Diabetes is common. Absence of awareness of hypoglycaemia may occur.

Musculoskeletal system, skin and temperature regulation

- Impaired responses to hypothermia (shivering and vasoconstriction occur at lower body temperatures). Shivering is less likely to be effective in restoring body temperature due to reduced muscle bulk. Hypothermia can occur quickly and will exacerbate bleeding by impairing coagulation.
- Osteoporosis means fractures are more likely, especially in elderly women.
- Skin tends to be thinner and less elastic and healing is impaired.
- Pre-existing mobility limitations and physical impairments may predispose to trauma.
- Pressure sores can develop quickly so contact with hard surfaces such as long boards and scoops should be kept to a minimum.

Capacity

- Some elderly patients may not have capacity to consent to treatment. In an emergency, acting in the patient's best interest usually means providing resuscitation unless clear evidence is produced to the contrary. However, determining whether resuscitation is appropriate should take into consideration any advanced directives applicable to the patient's current situation. Clearly in a life-saving situation, resuscitation should proceed where appropriate until a valid document is available.
- A Lasting Power of Attorney (LPA) may be granted by a competent patient to a person in the event of them losing capacity. However, life-saving or life-sustaining treatment can only be refused if the LPA was validly completed by the patient at a time when they had the capacity to do so.

Pharmacology in elderly patients

- Oral anticoagulants such as warfarin cause significant bleeding in trauma. Use of vitamin K may not always be applicable to the acute situation but warfarin reversal agents such as FFP and prothrombin complex concentrates (e.g. Beriplex, Octaplex) may be considered depending on the degree of bleeding and local guidelines.
- Polypharmacy: many elderly patients take several different medications which may influence the physiological response and actions of other drugs.
- Drug effects can be significantly different in the elderly.
- Volume of distribution falls due to reduced total body water and intravascular volume, and reduced cardiac output can slow drug distribution; plasma protein binding is reduced. This leads to higher relative plasma concentrations for IV drugs.
- Reduced cardiac output can slow distribution of drugs leading to a longer onset time for drug effect.
- Drug clearance is impaired by reduced glomerular filtration rate (GFR) and enzyme activity leading to prolonged action, plus accumulation of active metabolites.

Fractured neck of femur

Femoral fractures cause significant mortality in the elderly (up to 30% in some studies). Blood loss in a femoral fracture can reach 2 L. Pressure sores can develop quickly and care should be taken to reduce pressure on the heels and sacrum in particular. Fluid and electrolyte balance and ensuring normothermia are also important. Care pathways exist to improve management of elderly patients with femoral fractures. Early surgery has been shown to reduce the duration and severity of pain as well as the length of hospital stay. Analgesia should be titrated cautiously to pain, using opiates where needed. Femoral nerve blocks in the emergency department assist in pain control.

Cause and effect in trauma

Pre-existing illness may be the cause of trauma in the elderly: cardiac events, seizures, cerebrovascular events, mobility impairment, etc. can all precipitate trauma. Likewise, with a finite physiological reserve, the additional physiological stress of trauma can precipitate cardiac events, cerebral events, acute renal failure and many more life-threatening and life-limiting outcomes.

Burden on healthcare services

Elderly patients are more likely to suffer post-traumatic complications and have a slower recovery. Longer hospital stays are likely and long-term rehabilitation may be needed. This is a significant burden on healthcare services. The effects on individual patients may include loss of independence and isolation.

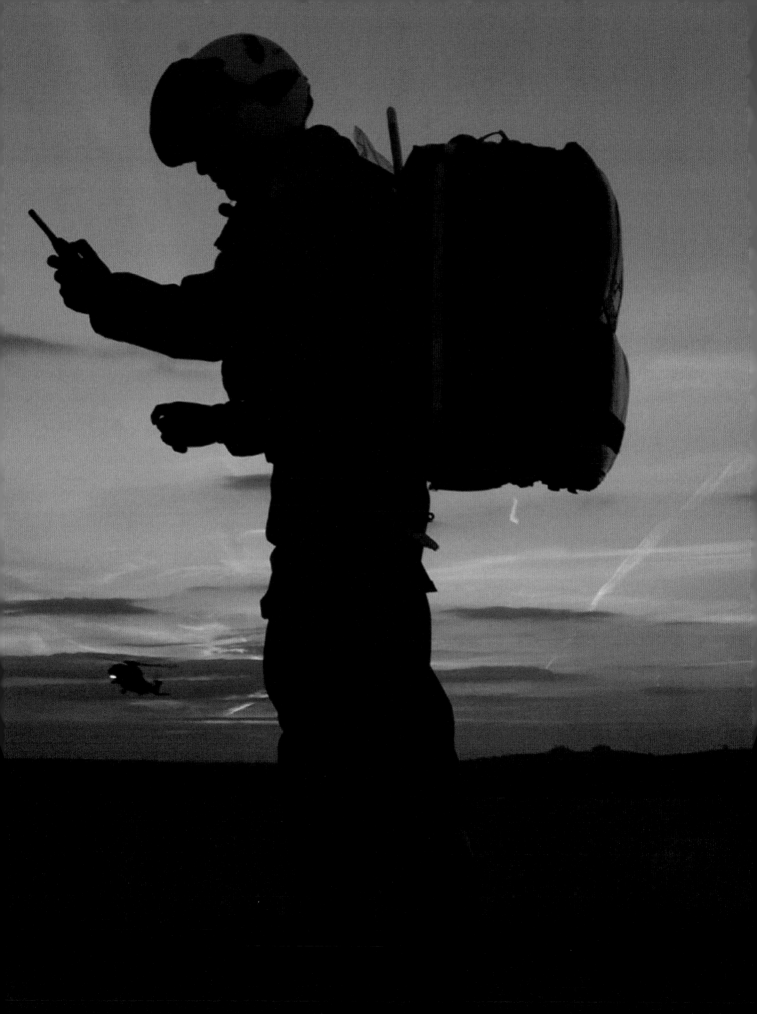

Practical skills in pre-hospital emergency medicine

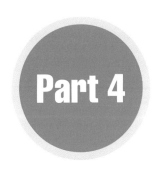

Part 4

Chapters

26 Anaesthesia in the pre-hospital environment

Figure 26.1 ABCDE management

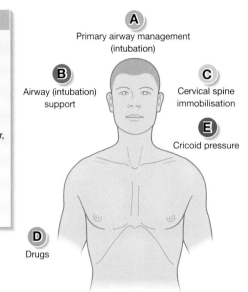

1 Prepare environment

- **Brief team** fully
- **Noise reduction:** team must be able to concentrate and to communicate effectively
- **360° access:** patient must be intubated with full access available; extrication from difficult areas must take place
- **Intubation position:** Patient on stretcher, procedure attempted at kneeling height, sun in front of A
- **Transport and transfer:** consider early (see 3)
- **Patient's dignity and privacy:** consider use of screens

A — Primary airway management (intubation)

B — Airway (intubation) support

C — Cervical spine immobilisation

E — Cricoid pressure

D — Drugs

2 Prepare monitoring

- **Full monitoring:** HR, BP, RR, SpO_2, $ETCO_2$, ECG
- **Back-up monitoring:** may be required in the field

3 Prepare transfer and transport

- **Consider early**
- **Communication:** consider pre-alerting receiving hospital of patient status pre- and post-intubation
- **Proximity to vehicle:** always intubate as close to road ambulance or helicopter as possible while taking into account clinical safety of patient

	A	B	C	D	E
Who?	Pre-hospital physician	HEMS/most experienced paramedic	Paramedic/EMT/ECA	AS/HEMS paramedic	Paramedic/EMT/ECA
Why?	Most senior clinical on scene	Intubation support	Immobilise C-spine while also managing polytrauma	Must be a senior clinician	Familiarity with cricoid pressure technique
What?	Airway management, pre-oxygenation, intubation (decision and process)	Setting up equipment, intubation 'kit dump'; right-hand man to intubator (**A**)	C-spine immobilisation, (including when collar removed)	Give anaesthetic and other drugs with correct timing	Apply cricoid pressure during intubation (technique checked and verbalised)

Figure 26.2 Limited space inside a helicopter

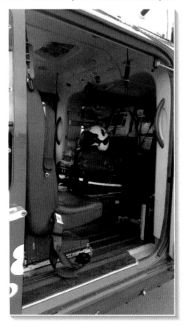

Figure 26.3 An RSI 'kit dump' used as a checklist on-scene

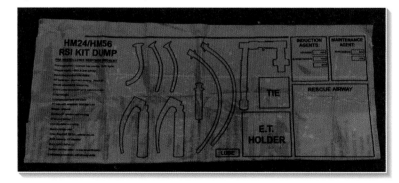

Pre-hospital Emergency Medicine at a Glance, First Edition. William Seligman, Sameer Ganatra, Timothy Parker and Syed Masud.
© 2018 John Wiley & Sons, Ltd. Published 2018 by John Wiley & Sons, Ltd.

Airway management is a priority in the resuscitation of a trauma patient and endotracheal intubation is the gold standard. Rapid sequence induction (RSI) describes the induction of general anaesthesia and subsequent endotracheal intubation. RSI is used in hospital for emergency anaesthesia only, since aspiration of stomach contents is a risk. However, since all pre-hospital anaesthesia is an emergency, RSI is indicated for all patients requiring anaesthesia in the field. The following issues must be taken into account when conducting pre-hospital anaesthesia.

Safety

Pre-hospital anaesthesia may be required on the road, in a field, or in the small confines of a house, whereas in-hospital anaesthesia is carried out in the controlled environment of an anaesthetic room. Pre-hospital anaesthesia must, therefore, have strict clinical governance, checklists and specific operating procedures.

Clinical complexity

Before in-hospital anaesthesia, patients undergo anaesthetic review weeks before surgery, and will always be starved before the procedure. In the pre-hospital phase, patients are often *in extremis*, critically ill with multiple injuries and unprepared for the anaesthetic procedure.

Operator-dependent

In hospital, the anaesthetic procedure will always be overseen by several doctors, including some who will be senior practitioners. If the procedure becomes complicated, support can be summoned quickly. In the field, the pre-hospital doctor may be the only physician on scene. The doctor will be required to carry out this procedure with limited help. It is imperative that the physician who practises anaesthesia in the field is of an appropriate grade with evidence of competency-based training. Practice and simulation training are pivotal to safe pre-hospital anaesthesia.

Transfer

After pre-hospital anaesthesia, the team must consider the issues of moving an anaesthetised and potentially unstable patient. The pre-hospital environment is not suitable for bulky equipment (e.g. multiple monitoring machines). The procedure of the move must be rehearsed and practised. When considering where to carry out the initial RSI, due thought must also be given to how the patient will be moved to the chosen transport vehicle. Movement must be kept to a minimum.

Transport

The team must consider the most appropriate mode of transport and the time involved in transporting the patient to the most appropriate hospital. Once the anaesthetised patient has been loaded into the chosen mode of transport, further assessment and clinical checks must be repeated.

Indications for pre-hospital anaesthesia

The decision to conduct pre-hospital anaesthesia is difficult and must be clearly indicated. Indications for pre-hospital anaesthesia can be stratified into the following main groups as guidance:

1 *Maintenance of the airway*: inability of patient to maintain effective airway (e.g. traumatic injury with facial fractures).
2 *Protection of the airway*: inability to protect airway, e.g. reduced conscious level or significant uncontrolled vomiting.

3 *Ventilation*: inability to ventilate appropriately, e.g. mechanical factors (fractured ribs, flail chest) or significant pre-morbid condition (asthma, chronic obstructive pulmonary disease).
4 *Oxygenation*: despite ventilation, the patient cannot oxygenate tissues adequately (e.g. haemorrhagic shock or poisoning).
5 *Clinical course*: the most difficult decision to make; requires experience to predict patient's pathway once delivered to hospital; pre-hospital RSI may save time if a patient's in-hospital management requires surgery; in patients with significant open injuries that are distressing and require significant in-hospital intervention, pre-hospital RSI may be indicated for humanitarian reasons; clinical course and humanitarian factors may be inextricably linked.

Once the decision for pre-hospital anaesthesia has been made, the following procedures must be strictly followed. The steps involved in RSI can be remembered using the **7Ps**:

1 **P**reparation: assess the patient for risk factors for difficult intubation and establish backup plans, attach monitoring; ensure the patency of at least one secure intravenous line; position the patient optimising 360° access; determine sequence of drugs and draw up into labelled syringes.
2 **P**re-oxygenation: administer high inspired fractions of oxygen for at least 3 minutes.
3 **P**re-treatment: administer drugs to mitigate adverse effects of intubation e.g. bronchospasm in patients with reactive airways disease, elevation of ICP, sympathetic discharge; the drugs to consider can be remembered using the mnemonic LOAD (**L**idocaine, for reactive airways disease or raised ICP; **O**pioid (fentanyl), when sympathetic responses should be blunted e.g. raised ICP, aortic dissection, intracranial haemorrhage, ischaemic heart disease; **A**tropine, for children who will receive suxamethonium; **D**efasciculation, before suxamethonium if patient has raised ICP).
4 **P**aralysis with induction: rapidly acting induction agent given followed by rapid push of neuromuscular blocker.
5 **P**ositioning: firm pressure over cricoid cartilage prevents regurgitation of gastric contents.
6 **P**lacement with proof: test jaw for flaccidity 45 seconds after paralytic agent given; intubate; confirm tube placement using – direct vision, Easi-Cap colourimetric carbon dioxide detector, bilateral breath sounds, absent epigastric sounds; discontinue cricoid pressure when cuff inflated.
7 **P**ost-intubation management: tape tube in place; administer maintenance sedation and paralysis.

An RSI 'kit dump' used as a checklist on-scene is shown in Figure 26.1.

Which drugs are used?

Induction agents

The ideal induction agent would have a rapid onset of action, short duration and a haemodynamically neutral profile. The choice of induction agent is governed by the clinical circumstance.

Paralysing agents

Suxamethonium is the most frequently used paralysing agent because it has the shortest onset of action (45 seconds) and short duration (6–8 minutes). It can occasionally cause life-threatening hyperkalaemia in already hyperkalaemic patients, i.e. those with burns/renal failure, and therefore *rocuronium* is sometimes used as an alternative. In addition, oxygen desaturation has been shown to occur later with use of rocuronium (most likely because muscle fasciculation occurs with suxamethonium), resulting in a longer safe apnoea time.

27 The emergency surgical airway

Figure 27.1 Cricothyroidotomy – step-by-step photo guide

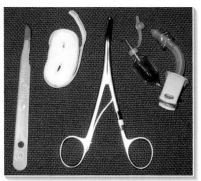

1. Kit required for emergency surgical airway (L to R): No. 20 scalpel; tube tie; dilators; cuffed size 6 ETT or tracheostomy tube

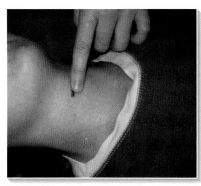

2. Identify the landmarks and mark with a pen

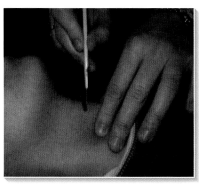

3. Stabilise larynx with left hand and make skin incision. Do not lose landmark

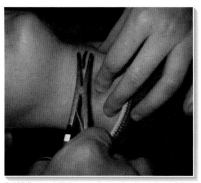

4. Whilst stabilising, make a single stab incision through cricothyroid membrane. Second operator should prepare dilator

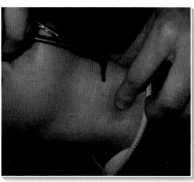

5. Dilate and rotate 90 degrees without letting go of landmarks

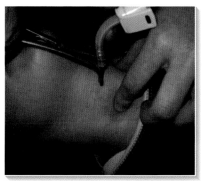

6. Insert tracheal device, secure and inflate cuff, check position

Figure 27.2 Surface anatomy

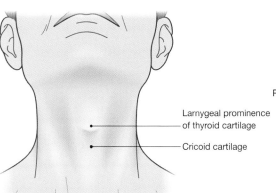

Larnygeal prominence of thyroid cartilage

Cricoid cartilage

Figure 27.3 Underlying anatomy

Note the cricothyroid membrane is palpable as a *springy* membrane in the depression just inferior to the laryngeal prominence of the thyroid cartilage

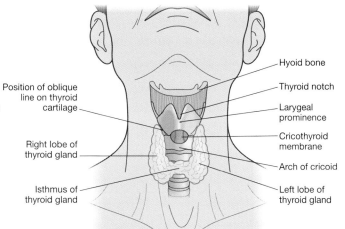

Position of oblique line on thyroid cartilage

Right lobe of thyroid gland

Isthmus of thyroid gland

Hyoid bone

Thyroid notch

Larygeal prominence

Cricothyroid membrane

Arch of cricoid

Left lobe of thyroid gland

Pre-hospital Emergency Medicine at a Glance, First Edition. William Seligman, Sameer Ganatra, Timothy Parker and Syed Masud.
© 2018 John Wiley & Sons, Ltd. Published 2018 by John Wiley & Sons, Ltd.

The failed airway drill

Timely and competent airway management is the top priority in any critically ill patient. Endotracheal intubation provides a definitive airway and is considered the gold standard for airway management. However, the austere environment of the pre-hospital setting and confounding factors such as complex facial trauma, severe oropharyngeal haemorrhage, and vomiting may reduce the likelihood of successful endotracheal intubation. Data have shown that up to 12.9% of all pre-hospital intubation attempts fail. Given the time-critical nature of airway management, the pre-hospital care practitioner must have a well-rehearsed standard operating procedure to ensure effective and expeditious ventilation and oxygenation.

Indications

Cricothyroidotomy is a rescue procedure, which is indicated in the 'can't intubate, can't ventilate' (CICV) situation where all alternative strategies of achieving a definitive airway have failed. The commonest indications include:

- severe maxillofacial trauma
- severe airway oedema (e.g. burns/anaphylaxis)
- an unstable C-spine
- an obstructing upper airway foreign body.

Contraindications

A common aphorism is that, given the incompatibility of loss of airway patency with life, there is no absolute contraindication to cricothyroidotomy. However, both lack of necessity (airway secured with less invasive means) and futility (for example, in tracheal transection with distal mediastinal retraction, or in the case of complicated laryngeal/cricoid cartilage fracture), are clear contraindications.

Relative contraindications include:

1 Loss of anatomical landmarks (e.g. due to obesity, substantial oedema, substantial surgical emphysema).
2 Children <10 years: poorly defined anatomical landmarks; greater incidence of laryngeal trauma; increased incidence of postoperative complications. *It is therefore recommended that paediatric cases initially receive needle cricothryoidotomy.*

Technique

Surgical cricothyroidotomy was first described by the French surgeon and anatomist Vicq d'Azyr in 1805. A total of 12 different methods have since entered practice, with use dependent largely on equipment availability and operator familiarity. Here, we describe the use of a modified three-step, two-person technique.

1 Preparation
- equipment ready (Figure 27.1)
- patient position – supine, neck in neutral alignment
- operator position – head-end of patient, side corresponding with operator's dominant hand
- trained assistant (paramedic)
- prepare surgical site (iodine spray).
2 Procedure
- Identify the cricothyroid membrane (Figures 27.2 and 27.3), fix skin, and make a 2–3 cm midline transverse incision with a No. 20 blade over the cricothyroid membrane. If surface anatomy is not readily identifiable, a midline vertical incision may be required to identify the cricothyroid membrane.
- Fix trachea with non-dominant hand and make a single horizontal stab through the cricothyroid membrane with finger over blade laterally to control depth of incision. Insert dilator into trachea and spread transversely, then rotate 90 degrees and dilate longitudinally. Ensure dilator is not removed from the opening in the cricothyroid membrane as bleeding will obscure view.
- Place cuffed 6.0 mm endotracheal tube inferiorly through spread dilators, inflate cuff and secure tube. Confirm placement with capnography/adjunctive measures.

Advantages

There are no significant differences in complication rates or the time required to perform any of the emergency surgical airway techniques. Operator familiarity and equipment availability are the key influences, and are controlled by use of standard operating procedure and frequent, rigorous drills for all members of the enhanced care team.

The major strength of the surgical airway, however, is the relative simplicity of the technique and the low equipment requirements, making this time-critical intervention as expeditious as possible. Compared with needle cricothyroidotomy, surgical techniques are at least as fast, if not faster, associated with higher rates of success at gaining front-of-neck airway access, and, critically, provide a definitive airway with optimum ventilation. Percutaneous transtracheal ventilation (PTV) following needle cricothyroidotomy delivers adequate oxygenation but, typically, does not allow effective expiration (small tube diameter limits flow), which may result in hypercapnoea. This is especially of concern in the head-injured trauma patient as hypercapnoea raises intracranial pressure. Further, PTV is associated with higher rates of barotrauma and pneumothorax.

Disadvantages

Emergency surgical airways do not kill patients; rather, it is reticence to perform the procedure that results in patient deaths. Both the psychological impact on the operator due to the invasiveness of the procedure and the relative infrequency of its implementation must be accounted for in the nature and frequency of training. Critically, this is a tactile procedure, as bleeding around the incision site will make subsequent visualisation of underlying structures extremely difficult; this must be factored into training with an intense focus on kinaesthetic learning.

The immediate complications are of primary concern to the pre-hospital practitioner as they must be addressed to ensure the airway is secured:

- failed/inadequate tracheal tube placement: misplaced incision with placement through thyroid membrane; creation of false passage; retrograde intubation; mainstem intubation
- tube occlusion with blood/vomitus
- haemorrhage/haematoma
- aspiration
- posterior tracheal/anterior oesophageal laceration.

28 Peripheral vascular access

Figure 28.1 A 16G large-bore cannula well-secured with tape to prevent dislodgement and loss of venous access during transit

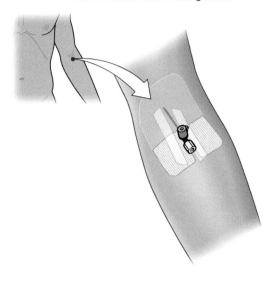

Figure 28.2 Venous cutdown, seldom used nowadays due to the development of more efficient methods of gaining vascular access, primarily intraosseous devices.

Source: *LifeART Collection images © 1989–2001 by Lippincott Williams & Wilkins, Baltimore, MD.*

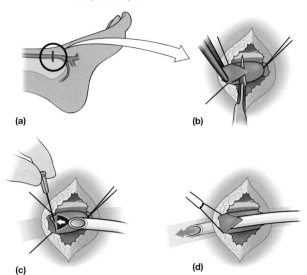

(a)   (b)

(c)   (d)

Figure 28.3 Cook® IO needle, manually-inserted device

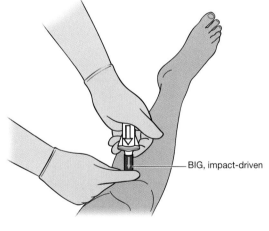

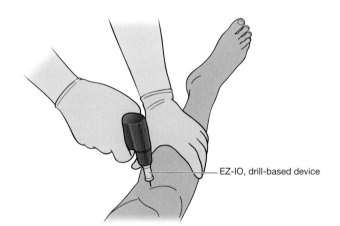

BIG, impact-driven

EZ-IO, drill-based device

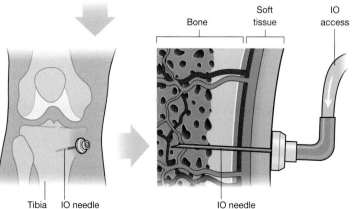

Bone   Soft tissue   IO access

Tibia IO needle   IO needle

Contraindications for IO access

Whilst IO needles are increasingly seen as the rescue option for patients in whom venous access is difficult, there are some contraindications, which may influence which site is chosen for access:

• Fracture or prosthesis in target bone
• IO access in the same limb in the previous 24–48 hours (including failed attempt)
• Overlying infection
• Inability to locate landmarks

Importance of circulatory access

Gaining vascular access promptly in the pre-hospital environment is imperative for fluid resuscitation and for the administration of intravenous drugs in critically unwell patients.

Venous access

Large-bore cannulae

Traditionally, circulatory access is gained by inserting a large-bore (14G–16G) cannula in the antecubital fossa. Suitable alternatives include the long saphenous vein, veins in the medial forearm, the dorsum of the hand and the feet. Ideally, two separate points of venous access should be obtained in different limbs, avoiding injured limbs and the arm ipsilateral to any chest injuries. In the case of suspected pelvic or inferior vena cava disruption, make sure that there is good access in place above the diaphragm.

Always maximise the chances of a successful first attempt by applying a venous tourniquet no more than 10 cm from the point of cannulation. Giving it time to work and having a trusted assistant hold the limb still will also help. If this fails, consider cannulating central veins: the subclavian, external jugular and femoral are options. This must be only attempted by enhanced care teams. Another option is to obtain small vein access and infuse 50–100 mL of fluid, keeping the tourniquet on, to dilate larger proximal veins which were previously inaccessible or less obvious.

If obtaining access is difficult, consider whether or not the patient absolutely requires immediate venous access in the field. Some casualties may not require urgent intravenous fluids or medication and so further attempts at siting a line can be carried out en route to hospital. In these cases, transport of the casualty to hospital should not be delayed for the sake of securing venous access. If cannulation is successful, it is critically important to secure the line effectively to safeguard against its disruption during evacuation and transport: apply two pieces of tape diagonally across the cannula and one horizontally; loop the giving set around the first webspace and back along the forearm, securing it with two more pieces of tape. Be mindful of sharps and dispose of them safely in a sharps bin.

Venous cutdown

A traditional, though nowadays seldom used, rescue technique when standard cannulation fails, is venous cutdown. This is where the vein is exposed surgically and a cannula is inserted into it under direct vision. The long saphenous vein at the ankle or groin or the basilic vein at the elbow are the usual sites of choice. As this is a surgical procedure that typically takes between 6 and 10 minutes, and due to the development of intraosseous devices and portable ultrasound machines, venous cutdowns are now rarely performed. However, it still retains a place in securing large bore access in a severely hypovolaemic patient.

If cutdown is a suitable intervention, the skin is cleaned, draped and local anaesthetic administered as required. A transverse skin incision is made, and a haemostat is used to carefully dissect down to the vein. The vessel is tied closed distally and transected proximally (venotomy). After dilating the vein, a cannula is introduced through the venotomy and is secured in place with a tie around the vein and cannula. Complications include haematoma, infection, and damage to surrounding structures (arteries and nerves). A quicker – and, arguably, safer – method is the mini-cutdown, wherein the vein is cannulated directly using a standard vascular catheter, without venotomy or ligatures. Though the cannula may not be as secure with this technique, it is a lot more efficient and more useful as a time-critical intervention.

A note on ultrasound

Portable ultrasound machines are increasingly being used in pre-hospital care, often to aid insertion of central and peripheral venous catheters. Although extra training is required in ultrasound, its use can dramatically increase rates of success in difficult cases while cutting down the incidence of complications.

Intraosseous devices

There are many factors which may render intravenous access difficult or even impossible to acquire: operator factors include poor technique or cumbersome personal protective equipment (e.g. hazardous materials suits); patient factors comprise extremes of age, venous shutdown (shock, cold), limb injuries and pre-existing vein damage (e.g. from intravenous drug use); environmental factors include difficult positioning of the patient and low light. In these situations, intraosseous (IO) access must be considered.

IO access was first used therapeutically in 1934 and reports throughout the 1940s confirmed the wide-ranging applicability of IO devices in delivering fluids, blood products, and medications to both adult and paediatric patients. However, the IO needle fell into disuse after the invention and rapid uptake of the venous catheter.

In recent years, there has been a resurgence in the use of IO devices, primarily in paediatric patients in whom vascular access is difficult, but who have easily identifiable bony landmarks. The advantage of IO in adults has now been proven and its use in the pre-hospital care environment is increasing. Several different devices exist but the unifying principle is that the tip of a needle is placed into the bone matrix, and infusions enter the systemic circulation via the bone marrow cavity. Devices may be manually inserted needles (e.g. Cook® IO needle), impact-driven (e.g. FAST-1 sternal IO device, BIG – bone intraosseous gun), or drill-based (EZ-IO): the latter two are particularly easy to insert and remove all uncertainty from the process (e.g. required depth of insertion).

The proximal tibia, sternum, and iliac crest are the three main preferred sites for IO access. Fractured limbs and orthopaedic implants should be avoided. Insertion should ideally be sterile but asepsis is adequate in the pre-hospital environment. Limb positioning and fixation is paramount here, and local anaesthetic should be given. Be vigilant for complications: extravasation of fluid, which may lead to compartment syndrome, fat embolism, fractures and osteomyelitis.

29 Chest techniques

Figure 29.1 Step-by-step thoracostomy using an innovative model

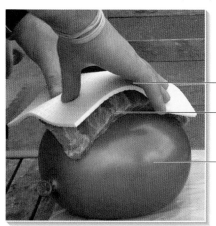

- Skin
- Ribs and intercostal muscles
- Pleura

1. Manually place three elements on one another to represent the chest wall with underlying lung

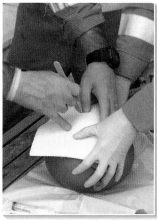

2. Identify an intercostal space by palpation and make a 1–1.5 inch incision with a size 20 scalpel into the thin domestic sponge simulating a subcutaneous incision

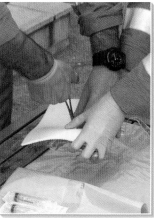

3. Using Spencer Wells forceps, blunt dissect through the intercostal muscles (rib spaces) until you reach the pleura. This will be felt when the forceps tips reach the balloon

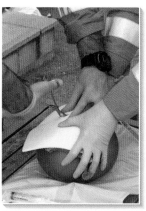

4. Firmly push against the pleura with the forceps until the balloon pops. Then by opening and closing the forceps increase the size of the intercostal hole so that one finger can pass through

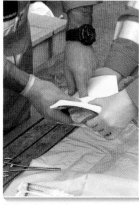

5. Simultaneously remove the forceps from the thoracostomy created as a finger is passed through

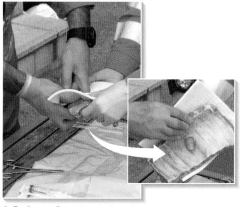

6. Perform a finger sweep to confirm the inside of the pleural cavity has been reached

Figure 29.2 Russell chest seal

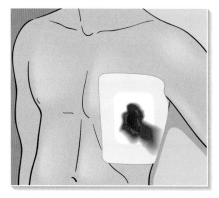

Figure 29.3 Asherman chest seal

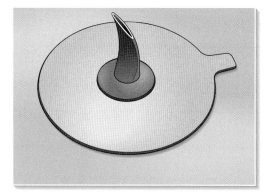

Pre-hospital Emergency Medicine at a Glance, First Edition. William Seligman, Sameer Ganatra, Timothy Parker and Syed Masud.
© 2018 John Wiley & Sons, Ltd. Published 2018 by John Wiley & Sons, Ltd.

Chest injury is a contributing factor in over half of all deaths from trauma. Mortality from an isolated chest injury is in the range of 4–8%. In the context of multiple organ involvement this rises to over 35%. It is therefore essential that pre-hospital care teams are able to assess rapidly and manage life-threatening chest injuries. In the pre-hospital care setting, it may be difficult to elicit and witness 'textbook signs' as injuries are often evolving and may not be fully established.

Thoracostomy

Thoracostomy involves making an incision in the pleural cavity. It may be used as the first step in the placement of a formal intercostal drain (tube thoracocentesis) or on its own to drain the pleura (simple thoracostomy). The advantages and disadvantages of each of the procedures is summarised in Table 29.1. Simple thoracostomy is performed more frequently in the pre-hospital setting.

The initial steps are the same in both procedures:

• personal protective equipment should be put on (sterile gloves; consider goggles)
• prepare all equipment ensuring sterility is maintained
• position the patient supine with the arm abducted as far as possible
• prepare the skin and place a drape over the area
• analgesia should be administered – lignocaine for local anaesthesia even in intubated patients and midazolam and ketamine in awake patients for procedural sedation
• using a scalpel, make a 2–3 cm incision along the line of the ribs in the fourth or fifth intercostal space in the mid-axillary line (Figure 29.4)
• blunt dissection above the inferior rib with Spencer Wells forceps to pass through the intercostal muscles
• push one finger into the pleural cavity to remove adhesions and clots and to feel whether or not the lung has re-expanded.

If simple thoracostomy is required, at this point the soft tissues should be left to fall back over the wound naturally. If a formal intercostal drain is to be placed, the drain is inserted to the same depth at the skin as the distance from the incision to the clavicle. The drain should then be sutured and taped in place.

Needle thoracocentesis

Traditional teaching is that needle thoracocentesis is the emergency management of tension pneumothorax. However, it must be

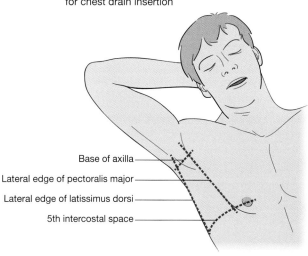

Figure 29.4 Surface anatomy depicting triangle of safety for chest drain insertion

Base of axilla
Lateral edge of pectoralis major
Lateral edge of latissimus dorsi
5th intercostal space

stressed that this is only a temporary measure; since it converts a tension pneumothorax to an open pneumothorax. It is, therefore, only performed by non-advanced pre-hospital care teams in peri-arrest situations before a more formal thoracocentesis is performed by enhanced care teams. The procedure is as follows: place a 14G cannula in the second intercostal space; mid-clavicular line. With differing body habitus, the 14G cannula may not be long enough to reach the pleural cavity. Although the procedure may be performed quickly, at best it removes the obstructive element to a shocked state. However, it does not facilitate lung re-expansion, and, as such, is significantly less useful than thoracostomy. Novel devices are emerging on the market to overcome some of the problems associated with the use of cannulae for this procedure, although thoracostomy is still more popular.

Chest seals for open chest wounds

Open chest wounds must be sealed in the pre-hospital phase to prevent an open pneumothorax from developing. A number of different chest seals exist but with similar properties:

• strong adherence to skin
• one-way valve to seal the hole and prevent air from entering chest cavity during inspiration, while allowing air/blood to pass out of the chest on expiration.

Table 29.1 Advantages and disadvantages of tube thoracocentesis and simple thoracostomy

	Tube thoracocentesis	Simple thoracostomy
Advantages	1 All physicians working in the pre-hospital phase should be familiar with this procedure from their in-hospital work 2 If placed correctly, it will save time once the patient arrives in hospital as the procedure will not need to be repeated	1 The lung can be felt to re-expand 2 It is possible to 're-finger' the thoracostomy if the patient deteriorates to rule out potential causes 3 Avoids the introduction of chest tubes in a non-sterile area 4 Avoids risk of re-tensioning as the system is not closed
Disadvantages	1 Increased movement in the pre-hospital phase may increase chances of the drain kinking, occluding, or being detached or moved out of position. Transport issues, e.g. decrease in amount of space on the helicopter, will make re-adjustments of the chest drain difficult 2 Once sutured in place, it becomes a closed system and can re-tension 3 Lung or clots can block the drainage holes within the chest drain tubing 4 The drain may kink inside the chest 5 The tubes connecting the drain to the collecting bag may kink or become blocked 6 Large airway leaks can rapidly fill the collecting system 7 Greater potential for infection	1 Theoretical risk of re-tension if the initial incision is blocked, i.e. the patient's arms or soft tissues occlude the hole when packaged.

30 Resuscitative thoracotomy

Figure 30.1 Clamshell thoracotomy step-by-step guide

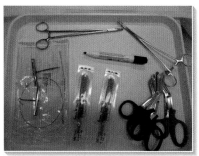

1. Equipment required for resuscitative thoracotomy

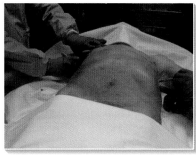

2. Start by making bilateral finger thoracostomies

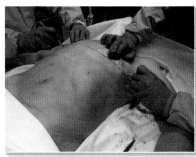

3. Join the thoracostomies with a transverse incision

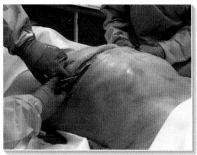

4. Using trauma scissors, cut from the thoracostomy, towards the sternum, above the level of the rib and following its curvature. Perform bilaterally

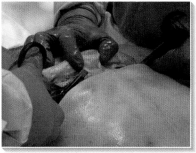

5. Divide sternum: trauma scissors are usually sufficient. However, if not, a Gigli saw may be required (see next picture)

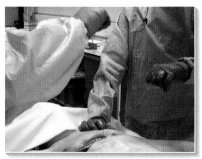

6. How to use a Gigli saw to divide the sternum

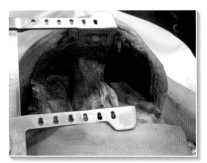

7. Open clam (using rib spreaders if available) to expose underlying anatomy

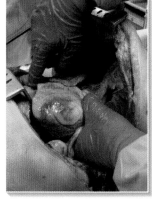

8. Open the pericardium, evacuate clots and deliver the heart to rapidly inspect for bleeding

Table 30.1 Control of cardiac haemorrhage ladder

Wound diameter	Occlusion technique	Caution
<1 cm	1. Finger 2. Gauze 3. Haemostatic gauze	Regularly reassess for haemostatic control, especially during transit
>1 cm	Foley catheter	Excessive traction can pull the catheter out and enlarge the primary wound
Refractory bleeding	Surgical staples	Rapid repair but only suitable for thick-walled ventricular wound
	Large suture	Take care not to occlude coronary arteries

Pre-hospital Emergency Medicine at a Glance, First Edition. William Seligman, Sameer Ganatra, Timothy Parker and Syed Masud.
© 2018 John Wiley & Sons, Ltd. Published 2018 by John Wiley & Sons, Ltd.

P re-hospital resuscitative thoracotomy was once seen by some as an 'heroic' intervention with a very poor outcome. However, emerging evidence has identified a specific subgroup of patients whose survival rates, with good neurological outcomes, approach 60%, if the thoracotomy is performed promptly and by the right team.

Indications

Based on the above, patients must meet each of the following strict consensus criteria for progression to pre-hospital resuscitative thoracotomy (RT):

- penetrating thoracic/epigastric injury
- in witnessed cardiac arrest (i.e. signs of life immediately following injury and preceding loss of output)
- attended within 10 minutes of loss of output
- tension pneumothorax excluded as cause.

Currently, any other indication for pre-hospital RT is insufficiently supported by evidence and therefore difficult to justify; however, there is increasing support for RT in proximal haemorrhage control following penetrating abdominal injury.

Contraindications

Absolute contraindications are based on futility of RT:

- medical cardiac arrest
- downtime more than 10 minutes.

Blunt trauma, severe head injury and damage to more than one body region are associated with very poor outcomes and also currently preclude RT. It should also be noted, however, that in practice, it is often difficult to establish precise time of loss of output and as such RT is often carried out when downtime is unclear.

Technique

The primary goal of RT is to gain rapid access to the heart to alleviate pericardial tamponade, control cardiac haemorrhage, and restore cardiac output.

Preparation

- Equipment ready (Figure 30.1).
- Patient position – supine, elbows extended, shoulders abducted.
- Trained assistant (enhanced care paramedic).
- Rapidly prepare surgical site (betadine spray).

Clam-shell thoracotomy

- Bilateral finger thoracostomies: abandon RT if this decompresses tension pneumothorax with resultant ROSC.
- Join thoracostomies with transverse incision.
- Using trauma scissors, cut from the thoracostomy towards the sternum bilaterally, above the level of the rib and following its curvature.
- Divide sternum: trauma scissors are often sufficient; if tough, may require Gigli saw.
- Open clam to expose underlying anatomy.
- Open pericardium, evacuate clots and deliver heart to inspect rapidly for bleeding.

Cardiac haemorrhage control

Cardiac defects must be identified and corrected with the minimum possible intervention. Wounds <1 cm diameter are usually successfully occluded with a finger or haemostatic gauze. Wounds >1 cm are sealed with a Foley catheter; this is advanced directly through the defect, the balloon inflated with ≤10 mL sterile water, and then withdrawn with careful traction to occlude the wound. This has the added benefit of permitting attachment of a giving set for direct, rapid volume, intracardiac blood transfusion (in the case of 'empty heart' following exsanguination). Refractory bleeding/large defects may be repaired with a large suture, although care must be taken to avoid occlusion of vital coronary arteries.

Restore cardiac output

Once venous return to the heart is restored, it may begin beating spontaneously. This may require initial or ongoing high quality internal cardiac massage, whereby an assistant provides direct thoracic aortic compression, while the heart is milked using a two-handed technique from apex to base at a rate of ~80 beats per minute. If the heart does not spontaneously begin beating after adequate blood resuscitation, a finger flick directly to the myocardium may deliver mechanical defibrillation; otherwise internal paddles or closure of the clamshell and use of standard external pads for electrical defibrillation is necessary.

Advantages

The clamshell technique for RT has a number of advantages, including its simplicity, its requirement for minimal non-specialist equipment, and its rapidity of access to the pericardium, typically within 2–3 minutes. It also provides excellent exposure for identification of bleeding points and ease of recognition of anatomy for non-surgeons. Additionally, the initial bilateral thoracostomies rapidly manage the key differential of obstructive shock due to tension pneumothorax, such that the more invasive clamshell may be easily abandoned if not indicated. The access obtained also permits lung lobar compression in the event of significantly bleeding pulmonary vasculature, and descending aortic compression for distal haemorrhage control.

Disadvantages

The relative scarcity of implementation of the technique and its immensely invasive nature combine to make RT extremely psychologically demanding for the pre-hospital practitioner; simply put, the first time it is used is the first time it is likely to have been practised. As ever in the acute stress of the pre-hospital environment, regular training and use of standard operating procedures to guide management helps to alleviate the human factors and facilitate delivery of gold standard emergency care.

Once cardiac output is restored, patients are likely to begin to haemorrhage from the open chest wound site, with bleeding most often problematic from the internal mammary and intercostal arteries; large vessel bleeding is usually managed with artery forceps. Furthermore, the patient will begin to regain consciousness, and will need anaesthesia, intubation and ventilation. Once stabilised, the patient should be promptly transferred to a major trauma centre with cardiothoracic facilities for definitive repair.

31 Pre-hospital ultrasound

Table 31.1 Diagnostic value of ultrasound

Major haemorrhage identification	• FAST (intra-abdominal fluid) • Chest (haemothorax) • Aortic aneurysm identification
Pulmonary injury	• Pneumothorax • Haemothorax • Pulmonary contusion
Cardiac injury	• Pericardial effusion • Cardiac muscle injury
Fluid status	• Cardiac tamponade • Cardiac ventricular contractility and size • Inferior vena cava status
Traumatic cardiac arrest – identification of potential causes	• FAST (intra-abdominal bleed/hypovolaemia) • Chest – pneumothorax • Cardiac tamponade • Fluid status
Cranial injury	• Raised intra-cranial pressure
Bone ultrasound	• Fracture identification

Table 31.2 The use of ultrasound as a procedural aid

Vascular access	• Femoral vein access • Central venous access
Nerve blocks	• As an adjunct to traditional analgesia
Checking placement of endotracheal tubes	• To ensure endotracheal rather than oesophageal intubation
Insertion of surgical airway	• Identification of cricothyroid membrane

Figure 31.1 Areas that are scanned as part of the e-FAST scan

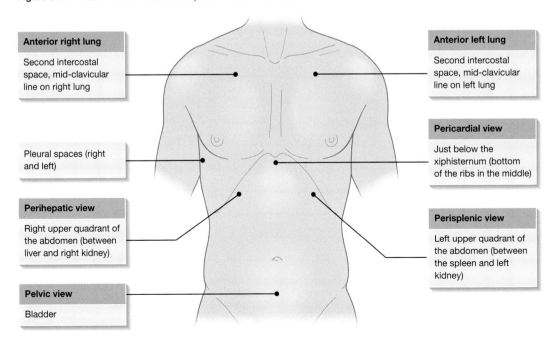

Anterior right lung

Second intercostal space, mid-clavicular line on right lung

Anterior left lung

Second intercostal space, mid-clavicular line on left lung

Pericardial view

Just below the xiphisternum (bottom of the ribs in the middle)

Pleural spaces (right and left)

Perihepatic view

Right upper quadrant of the abdomen (between liver and right kidney)

Perisplenic view

Left upper quadrant of the abdomen (between the spleen and left kidney)

Pelvic view

Bladder

Pre-hospital Emergency Medicine at a Glance, First Edition. William Seligman, Sameer Ganatra, Timothy Parker and Syed Masud.
© 2018 John Wiley & Sons, Ltd. Published 2018 by John Wiley & Sons, Ltd.

Ultrasound has been used as a diagnostic aid in medicine for over 50 years. In the past 20 years, ultrasound has moved from being a specialist imaging technique provided by radiologists and cardiologists to a diagnostic tool used in diverse clinical arenas, including anaesthesia, intensive care, gastroenterology, chest medicine and emergency medicine. The use of ultrasound by non-radiologists is known as 'focused ultrasound' and is deployed to answer specific clinical questions rather than being a detailed study of a specific anatomical region.

There is great potential benefit for the use of ultrasound in pre-hospital emergency medicine. The most valuable potential benefit is in making a diagnosis earlier and so facilitating timely definitive care. Ultrasound may also be used in pre-hospital procedures including gaining vascular access, nerve blocks and confirming placement of intraosseous and endotracheal tubes. The potential uses of ultrasound within the pre-hospital environment are highlighted in Tables 31.1 and 31.2.

Focused assessment with sonography in trauma (FAST scan)

Many trauma patients have injuries that may not be apparent in the primary survey. Significant bleeding into the peritoneal, pleural or pericardial spaces may occur without obvious warning signs. In order to reduce both mortality and morbidity from trauma, it is necessary to recognise potential areas of blood loss and bleeding as early as possible in the resuscitation of patients. The purpose of the now widely used FAST scan is to identify rapidly free fluid (usually blood in the context of trauma) in the peritoneal, pericardial or pleural spaces, suggesting visceral injury and occult blood loss as a cause of hypovolaemic shock.

The FAST exam, as originally described, looks at both the abdomen and the pericardium. Additional views added to the FAST exam looking for evidence of pneumothorax and haemothorax, commonly referred to as the extended FAST or e-FAST, can extend the usefulness of ultrasound in trauma care. The areas that are scanned as part of the e-FAST scan are shown in Figure 31.1. They reflect the dependent areas where fluid (blood) is likely to distribute. The FAST scan should not be undertaken prior to patient extrication as this will delay extrication and prevent other more critical interventions. Once the patient has been extricated, the FAST scan can be undertaken with the patient supine, ideally while en route to a receiving facility to minimise delays on scene.

Ultrasound as a procedural aid

Ultrasound imaging is used commonly in the hospital setting to aid identification of peripheral and central veins for cannulation.

Complications of central venous cannulation are common, even under ideal conditions. In the pre-hospital setting, where obtaining venous access is more likely to be difficult, there is therefore a role for ultrasound. Ultrasound has been shown to reduce the number of attempts required for successful central cannulation, to reduce failure rates and to reduce the time to successful placement. The use of ultrasound also reduces the likelihood of complications.

Practicalities of ultrasound in the pre-hospital environment

Ultrasound machines are becoming lighter, tougher, cheaper and produce increasingly clear images. There are now battery-powered machines that can be used in the rugged pre-hospital environment. However, there are a number of issues that may influence a pre-hospital care practitioner's decision on whether or not to use ultrasound:

1 Practical implementation:
  • Images which are taken in the pre-hospital environment should be presented to the receiving team in hospital for their own information and interpretation. This can be difficult.
  • Training: there are as yet no competencies or minimal training records that have to be completed before a practitioner can use ultrasound in PHEM.
  • Operator-dependent: as with any other diagnostic test that requires interpretation, ultrasound is only as good as its operator and his/her interpretation of the images.
  • Timing issues: should the scan be carried out in the primary survey or before packaging, or even while transporting the patient? This debate has led to concerns that ultrasound may delay on-scene times further and slow down the patient's journey to definitive care.

2 Environment:
  • Noise: in the controlled environment of the outpatient department, ultrasound is carried out in a sterile, quiet and dark area. Light can be a major barrier to interpretation of ultrasound images. In bright sunlight, for instance, scans can be very difficult to interpret. Scanning under a blanket or use of a specific screen cover for the machine may help. An alternative location for scanning, for example inside an ambulance, may be required for accurate interpretation of scans.
  • Movement: movement artefact can significantly degrade the quality of ultrasound images. To see accurate images, the patient and the operator need to be as still as possible at all times. Transportation of patients in either a land-based ambulance or a helicopter will make this particularly difficult and should be taken into consideration when deciding when best to scan without delaying transportation of the patient.

32 Packaging

Figure 32.1 Typical restricted conditions in the back of a HEMS helicopter.
Source: *By Sandstein (Own work) [CC BY-SA 3.0 (http://creativecommons.org/licenses/by-sa/3.0)], via Wikimedia Commons.*

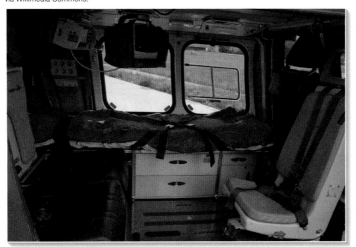

Box 32.1 Minimal movement, maximum safety

• Use of a scoop stretcher reduces total rotation of the patient at the scene and in hospital, minimising the chance of clot disruption and hypotension, as well as spinal cord damage.

• Each movement has the potential to cause more pain to the patient and so unnecessary movements should be avoided. Further, in the unconscious patient, significant rotation can allow for secretions and the tongue to fall back, disrupting the airway.

Figure 32.2 Comparing total rotation with logroll to total using scoop and minimal movement

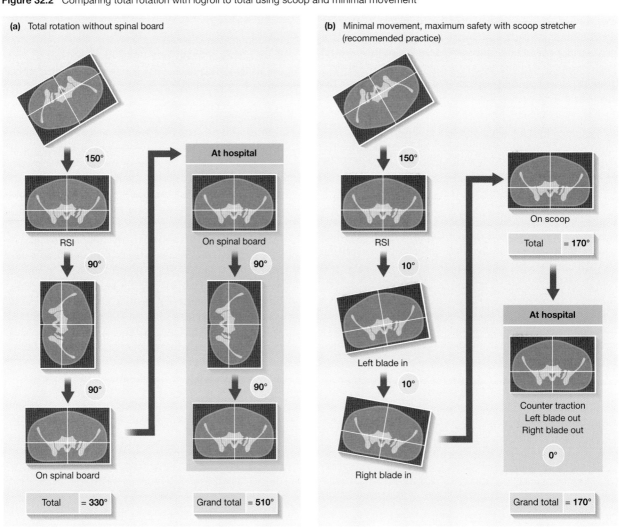

(a) Total rotation without spinal board

150° → RSI → 90° → On spinal board → 90° → On spinal board
Total = 330°

At hospital
150° → On spinal board → 90° → 90°
Grand total = 510°

(b) Minimal movement, maximum safety with scoop stretcher (recommended practice)

150° → RSI → 10° → Left blade in → 10° → Right blade in

On scoop
Total = 170°

At hospital
Counter traction
Left blade out
Right blade out
0°

Grand total = 170°

What is packaging?

Innovation in pre-hospital care on-scene and in critical care at the hospital has been impressive, but the journey from the scene to the hospital remains a limiting factor. Treatment in the back of a helicopter or an ambulance can be impeded and the ability of teams to alter their management plan while in transit is highly limited. Therefore, it is crucial to ensure that the casualty is optimally prepared for transport – this is the aim of packaging.

Patient-oriented packaging

Minimal movement, maximum safety

Immobilisation is key in packaging. It minimises serious pain (using bone splinting), serious morbidity (spinal cord injury) and mortality (dislodgment of formed clots). *Splinting limb fractures* minimises pain by eliminating unnecessary movement at fracture sites. Bringing bones back into anatomical alignment precludes the mobile ends of fractured bones from damaging blood vessels, causing further haemorrhage, and also reduces the area into which any torn blood vessels can bleed. *'Clot and cord' management* can be grouped together, as the measures taken to prevent spinal cord damage also minimise clot disruption. Traditionally in the UK, spinal cord immobilisation involves the use of a cervical collar and blocks secured to a rigid spinal board with the patient log-rolled onto and off the board. However, in a consensus statement from the Faculty of Prehospital Care in 2013, Moss *et al.* (2013) have stated that the long spinal board should be used only as an extrication device, and not for patient transfer to hospital. While safeguarding against cord injury, the log-rolling required to move the patient onto and off the board risks causing further haemorrhage from disrupting the clots formed naturally (typically over a period of 10 minutes) by the patient's coagulation cascade after trauma. Indeed, in the resuscitation room, blood pressure characteristically falls at three points: log-rolling off the spinal board, log-rolling for spinal examination, and log- rolling when preparing the patient for CT scan.

The principle of a single movement early on in the patient's care should be adopted with the intention of avoiding any unnecessary movement in order to promote haemostasis. Moss *et al.* made three key recommendations to this end, all of which are increasingly becoming standard clinical practice:

1 A *scoop stretcher* should be used instead of a spinal board, which reduces total rotation of the patient over the course of evacuation and transfer to a hospital bed from around 510° to 170° (Figure 32.2).

2 The casualty should be immobilised with '*skin-to-scoop*'. This means that all clothing should be removed at the incident scene in order to preclude unnecessary handling in hospital to gain full exposure for a secondary survey. However, it should be noted that skin-to-scoop compromises patient dignity and risks hypothermia. It should only be carried out for those with multiple injuries or shocked patients, not those with isolated fractures, including an isolated suspected C-spine fracture.

3 In the resuscitation room, examination of the patient's back should be carried out after removal of the scoop stretcher, enabled by *minimal (10°) tilt*, not a full log-roll.

Furthermore, if transfer to a point of definitive care is likely to take more than 45 minutes, the use of a *vacuum mattress* should be considered to avoid pressure-related skin and soft tissue damage. Preventing this would otherwise require regular extra handling of the patient, which would be harmful and impractical in transit.

Optimisation of clinical condition before transfer

Given that only very limited interventions can be carried out while in transit, the patient must be made as stable as possible before entering the vehicle or aircraft. The patient's airway must be secure, with intubation carried out if indicated before transit, and haemodynamic status optimised. Further cytokine release must be minimised as it leads to a widespread immune response, systemic vasodilation and hypotension. Therefore, further tissue damage must be prevented through immobilisation and appropriate fluid resuscitation. Hypothermia must be avoided in order to prevent acidosis and coagulopathy (lethal triad of trauma). This is particularly important in the light of skin-to-scoop practice and bubble wrap is commonly used for this in the field.

Provider-oriented packaging

Packaging from the perspective of the care provider relates to the logistics of transporting the patient and any accompanying passengers to hospital, and the handover of that patient to definitive care.

Equipment

Pre-hospital care practitioners must make sure that all treatment and monitoring kit is secure during evacuation and transport. Wires, lines and leads should be checked to be functioning and free from entanglement before entering the vehicle and re-checked once inside. One intravenous access point must be easily accessible during transit in case fluids or medications need to be infused.

Passengers

Although space is very restricted in the back of an ambulance or a helicopter, pre-hospital teams may have to transport passengers alongside the patient in certain situations. Police and firearm specialists may be required for tactical operations for the protection of the ambulance crew and potentially the patient in instances of gang warfare, for example. Though relatives are, in general, discouraged from accompanying the patient to hospital, in the case of a distressed child, the presence of a calming parent may facilitate decisive treatment and improve patient outcome. All passengers must be fully briefed about the situation prior to transit and be guided in terms of how to behave while in the ambulance or helicopter. The patient, if conscious, should also be briefed for the sake of reassurance and cooperation.

Handover

It is the responsibility of the pre-hospital care practitioner to lead the transfer of the patient to a hospital bed in a controlled manner. To avoid further unnecessary handling, the findings of any back examination should be relayed to the receiving team and written in the notes.

33 Handover

Figure 33.1 Handover form

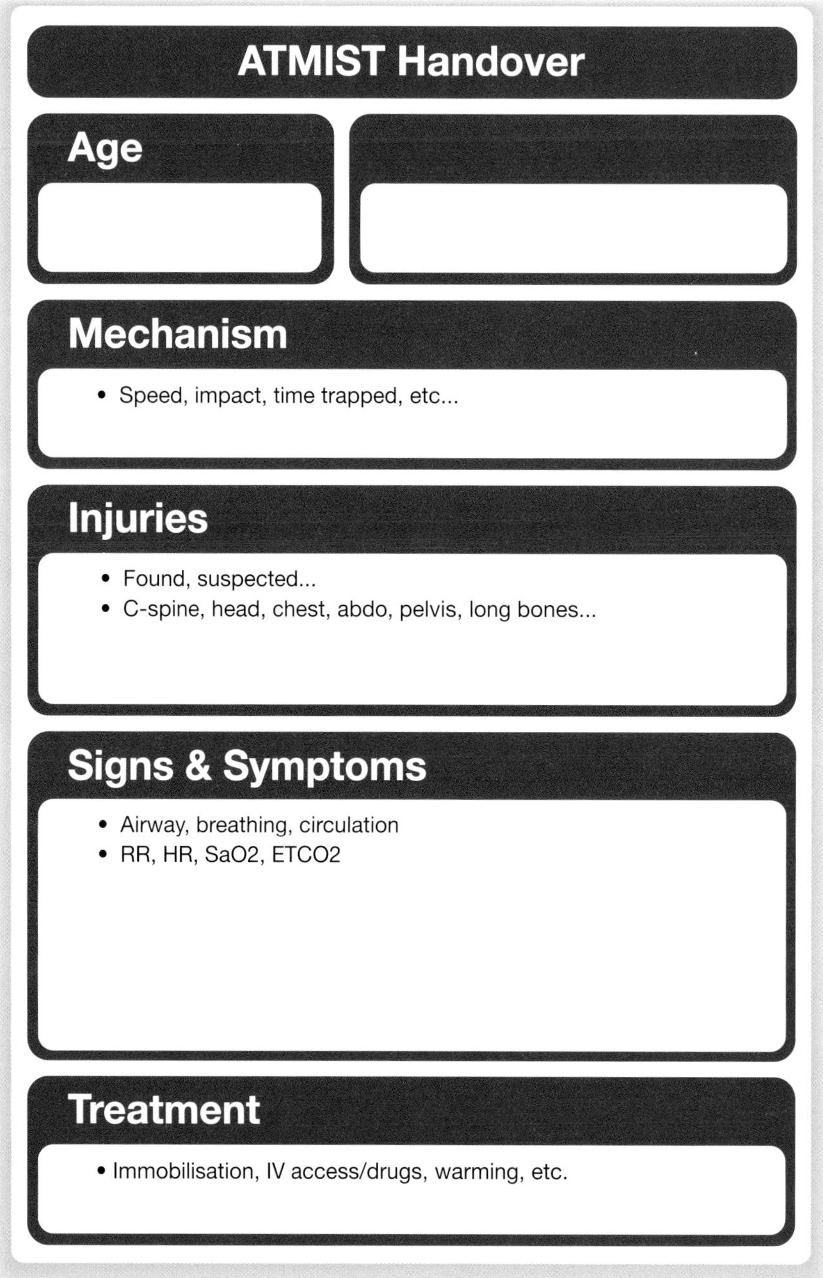

ATMIST Handover

Age

Mechanism

- Speed, impact, time trapped, etc...

Injuries

- Found, suspected...
- C-spine, head, chest, abdo, pelvis, long bones...

Signs & Symptoms

- Airway, breathing, circulation
- RR, HR, SaO2, ETCO2

Treatment

- Immobilisation, IV access/drugs, warming, etc.

Pre-hospital Emergency Medicine at a Glance, First Edition. William Seligman, Sameer Ganatra, Timothy Parker and Syed Masud.
© 2018 John Wiley & Sons, Ltd. Published 2018 by John Wiley & Sons, Ltd.

As pre-hospital care teams now provide a wide range of interventions, it is more important than ever that information is handed over effectively to the Emergency Department team. With critically ill or unstable patients, this transfer of information and care must be performed rapidly. However, it must be completed in a manner that ensures that all team members understand the patient's pre-hospital journey. Considerable communication skills are required, as well as knowledge of human factors, to ensure that the handover process is as effective as possible. With verbal communication accounting for just 20% of the transfer of information, it must be precise, clear, accurate and incorporate effective non-verbal techniques.

Preparing for handover and the pre-alert

Handover is a skill that should be approached in just the same way as a clinical procedure. As such, the pre-hospital team must undertake significant preparation before commencing handover in hospital. Handover starts, however, with a telephone pre-alert to the receiving hospital using a standard format e.g. SBAR (situation, background, assessment, recommendation). This message should be planned and rehearsed before transmitting. An example pre-alert message is shown below:

I am Dr X with the HEMS team.
This is an adult trauma, code red.
Mechanism of injury: 24-year-old female who has been hit by a car travelling at 25 miles per hour and bullseyed the windscreen.
Injuries: initial GCS was 3. Her legs were splayed.
Management: she has been RSI'ed on scene but she remains hypotensive and tachycardic.

Assessment: my assessment is that she has a severe traumatic brain injury as well as a pelvic fracture with vascular injury.
Conveyance: ETA 10 minutes. We require adult trauma team and code red protocol.
Repetition: would you like to repeat the information back to me?

How to give an effective handover

Handover must be given in a specific way structured to maximise the effectiveness of communication. Handover should take place in the resuscitation room with all members of the receiving team present. Handover must not take place while moving and should not be given to a single or selected members of the receiving team. The receiving team should be silent during handover. The recommended sequence is as follows:

1 The pre-hospital team states whether or not the patient has any urgent needs. If so, these are addressed immediately.
2 If not, the patient is transferred onto the hospital trolley: the scoop should be removed in a controlled manner by traction and counter-traction and not a full log roll.
3 The pre-hospital team delivers the handover in the following order:
- name and age of patient
- time of injury
- mechanism of injury
- injuries suspected from top to toe
- pre-hospital interventions provided
- summary.

After handover, the pre-hospital team should complete any required paperwork and restock used equipment. They should not be involved in the ongoing management of the patient unless specifically asked to do so by the hospital Team Leader.

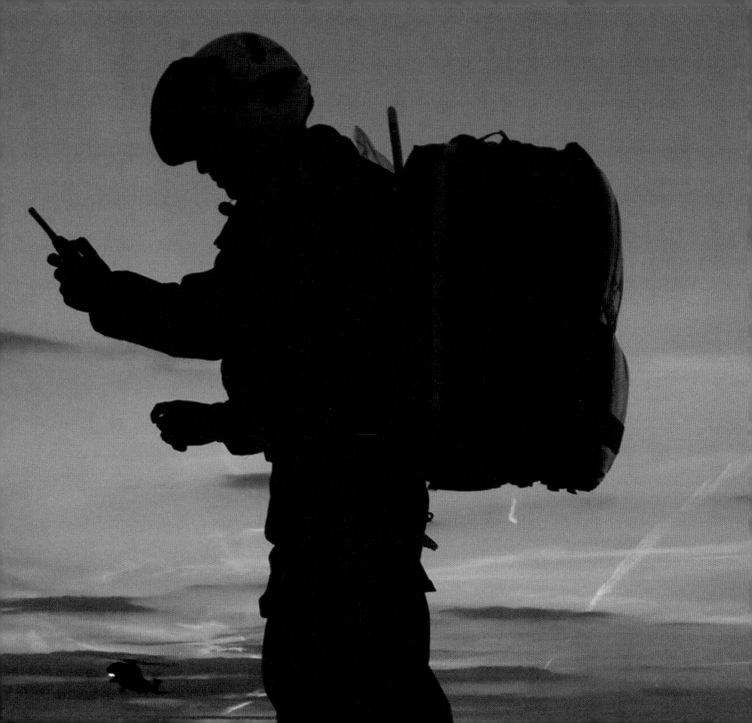

Management of complex problems

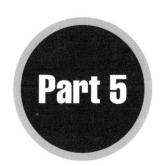

Part 5

Chapters

34 Major incidents

Figure 34.1 A major incident   Source: *Hughes T. and Cruickshank J.* Adult Emergency Medicine at a Glance *(2011). Reproduced with permission of John Wiley & Sons.*

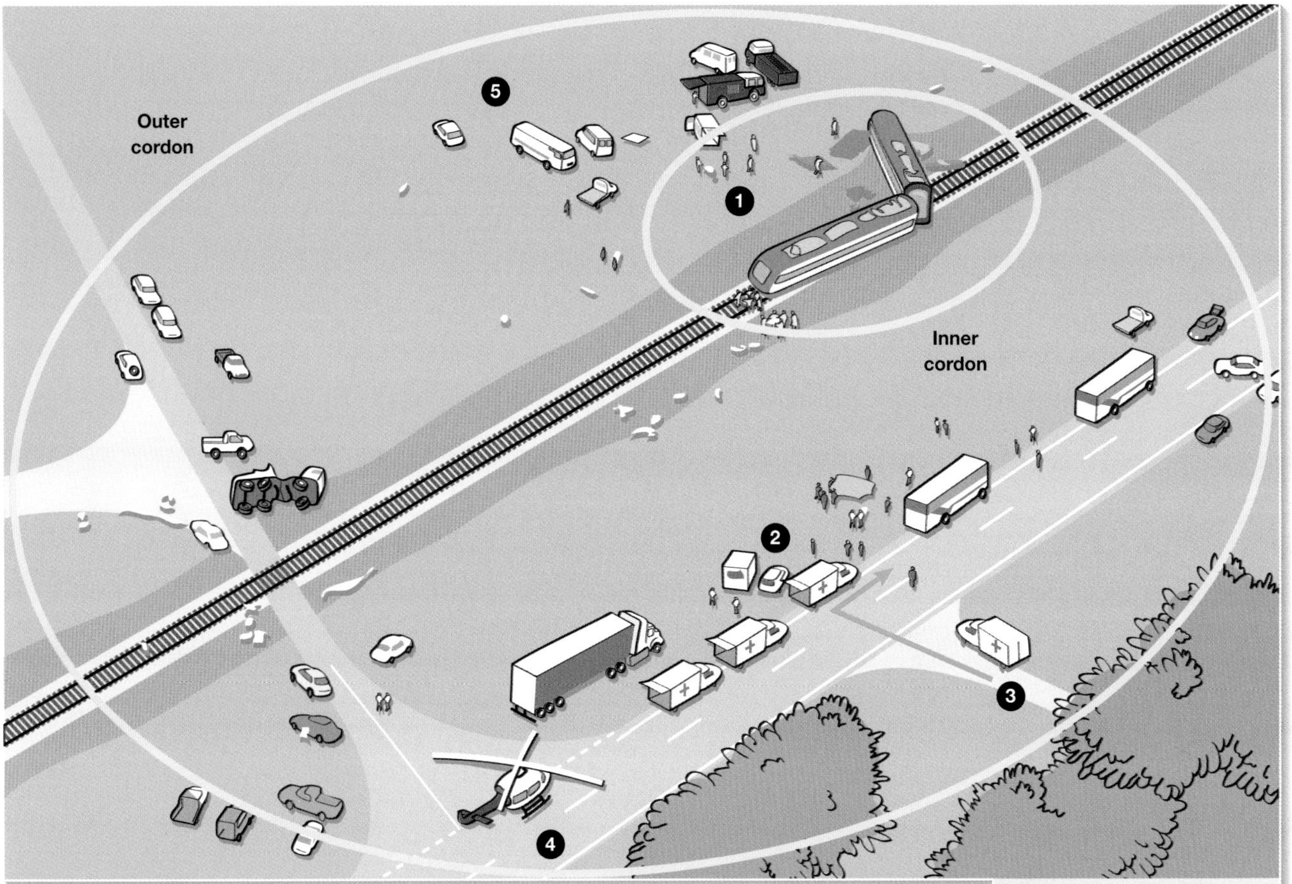

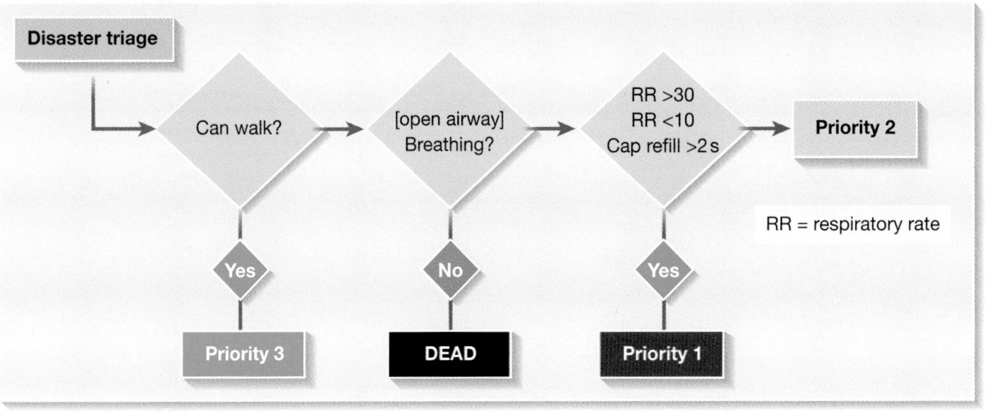

Outer cordon

Inner cordon

Disaster triage

Can walk? → [open airway] Breathing? → RR >30 RR <10 Cap refill >2 s → **Priority 2**

RR = respiratory rate

Yes → **Priority 3**

No → **DEAD**

Yes → **Priority 1**

1 Forward triage point
2 Casualty clearing station
3 Ambulance loading
4 Helicopter landing site
5 Incident control post

Pre-hospital Emergency Medicine at a Glance, First Edition. William Seligman, Sameer Ganatra, Timothy Parker and Syed Masud.
© 2018 John Wiley & Sons, Ltd. Published 2018 by John Wiley & Sons, Ltd.

A major incident is defined as any incident where the location, number, severity or type of live casualties requires extraordinary resources. Pre-hospital care practitioners will often be the first to respond to major incidents and it is therefore essential that they are familiar with the principles of managing major incidents as well as with local major incident protocols and policies.

Declaring a major incident and initial management priorities

The first priority of a pre-hospital care team on arrival at an incident that they suspect requires extraordinary resources is to declare a major incident. This allows Emergency Operations Centres to coordinate a response appropriate to the incident. A standard mnemonic used for notifying a major incident is METHANE:

Major incident declared
Exact location
Type of incident
Hazards present and potential
Access
Number and severity of casualties
Emergency services present and requested

After declaring a major incident, the priorities for initial management include: **C**ommand, **S**afety, **C**ommunication, **A**ssessment, **T**riage, **T**reatment, **T**ransport. Further details on what is involved in each of these priorities follows.

Safety at major incidents

The police force has overall primacy at major incidents. On arrival at the scene, the police will cordon off the incident. The inner cordon contains the immediate area around the incident, and the outer cordon contains all the emergency services attending the incident. The Fire and Rescue Service, on arrival, will check that the area is safe before allowing healthcare personnel access to casualties in the inner cordon.

Establishing the infrastructure

If assuming the role of Major Incident Commander (the most senior physician on-scene), one of the key responsibilities is to develop the major incident infrastructure ensuring key roles and places are clearly defined. This must be done in consultation with the Ambulance Incident Commander (often the enhanced care team paramedic). Without an effective infrastructure, chaos ensues and patient management is affected. Key points in the infrastructure include:

1 Establishing a rendez-vous point. This is the point to which all emergency services personnel will be sent. It should not, therefore, be sited in the middle of the scene.

2 Establishing designated access and egress routes. These must be carefully selected to ensure there are no obstructions to access or egress.

3 Establishing the ambulance parking point. This is where ambulances will wait to be called forward to collect a patient. This area must be strategically located to be on the access route without cluttering the scene.

4 Establishing the casualty clearing station. This is the position to which casualties will be brought for treatment prior to transport. This should be located next to the ambulance loading point to ensure effective conveyance of patients from the incident to definitive in-hospital care.

5 Ambulance loading point. See above. This is where patients are loaded into waiting ambulances.

6 Joint Emergency Services Control Centre (JESCC). This is where all the emergency service command vehicles are located and where regular tri-service meetings take place.

7 A log in which all actions taken in the management of the response are recorded must be started. Photos should be included where appropriate. This can be recorded on a mobile telephone initially and later transcribed. This is essential in providing evidence at inquests, which may take place several years after the incident.

Triage

Triage should only begin once the infrastructure is in place and scene safety ensured. Triage does not mean treatment and it is essential to complete primary triage before treatment begins. The triage sieve is shown diagrammatically in Figure 34.1, but essentially patients are categorised according to the following questions:

1 Can they walk? If so, P3.
2 Are they breathing? If not, dead.
3 Is their respiratory rate greater than 30, less than 10 or do they have capillary refill times of greater than 2 seconds. If so, P1, otherwise P2.

Patients should be labelled with clearly visible cards showing their priority status. Remember, however, that triage is a dynamic process. A patient's condition may improve or deteriorate and so there must be an opportunity for recategorisation. This often occurs once casualties reach the casualty clearing station and undergo secondary triage.

Conclusion

Fortunately, major incidents in the UK happen infrequently. However, pre-hospital care teams must be prepared to respond effectively at any time. Regular training and tri-service exercises should be carried out frequently to prevent difficulties at real incidents. Once on-scene, the key priority for pre-hospital care teams is to establish the infrastructure. History shows that where this has been implemented effectively, even hugely complex and evolving scenes (e.g. at Aldgate Station on 7 July 2005), can be cleared within a short period of time.

35 Expedition medicine

Figure 35.1 Expedition preparation

Altitude

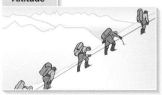

Polar

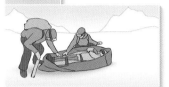

Desert

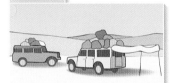

Jungle

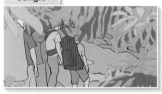

The medic and the team

- **The expedition leader (EL)** – the EL will have experience in the environment. There may be a local guide also. The EL and the medic have an important relationship and should be a united unit. Work out any disagreements behind closed doors
- **Introductions** – make individual contact with the team members via email or phone
- **Medical questionnaire** – encourage full disclosure, emphasise confidentiality and explain that you are there to primarily facilitate their trip, not to stop people from going
- **Professionalism** – maintaining professional objectivity while remaining a friendly active team player is a tricky balance
- **Confidentiality and candour** – the team must feel free to approach you. Consider a time that you will hold a daily clinic
- **Documentation** – document your consultations as normal. Provide GP letters as needed
- **Small group dynamics** – expect strange reactions to the isolation and fatigue

Communications

- **Ensure effective 'comms' and understand limitations of each type** – reliance on mobile phones is unwise. Satellite phones, a must for the majority of expeditions, still require a view of the sky
- **Understand** – the local and international emergency channels and practice concise distress calls.
- **Brief team** – about messages home and social media if there is a serious incident

The expedition medic

- **Training** – take an expedition medicine course to learn, network and get advice
- **Payment/expenses** – be clear. You are either a paying client (i.e. no medical duties beyond 'Good Samaritan' acts) or you are employed as the expedition medic
- **Indemnity** – always discuss your plans with your provider. There may be an extra fee
- **The medical team** – gather the medical team together as early as possible

The expedition medical kit

- **Ready-made** – may be provided. Readymade kits are available but expensive. Consider kit carefully and be realistic about what care can be provided
- **Drugs** – doctors can write a private prescription in any pharmacy but now must provide evidence that the medication is not for their own use
- **Controlled drugs (CDs)** – taking CDs across borders is often more trouble than it is worth, especially for smaller, low-risk trips. Discuss with the MHRA (Medicines Healthcare Products Regulatory Agency)

Medical evacuation (medevacs)

- **The patient** – is likely to need to be moved by land initially. A helicopter landing site may have to be created (twice the diameter of its blades) and a weather report given, including cloud levels and wind
- **Medical insurance** – a medical report will be requested. Have low expectations on how rapid the evacuation will be
- **Medevacs** – are difficult for the whole team

Pre-hospital Emergency Medicine at a Glance, First Edition. William Seligman, Sameer Ganatra, Timothy Parker and Syed Masud.
© 2018 John Wiley & Sons, Ltd. Published 2018 by John Wiley & Sons, Ltd.

Types of expedition

• Solo/pairs – often require remote advice, a supply of basic medical equipment and some training.
• Small group – may be static (e.g. scientific teams, or mobile on a specific route such as charity treks), normally one medic.
• Large group – often require more than one medic and a support team (e.g. gap year projects).
• Remote area endurance races – serious undertakings with large medical teams.

Preparing for the expedition

• Personal medical kits – simple first aid kits should be carried by all members including a supply of their own regular medication. The main medical kit is for emergencies.
• Dental checks – dental issues are very common and can be a disaster. Encourage an early check-up, including you.
• Vaccinations/antimalarials – be clear on current advice and lead by example. Websites such as www.nathnac.org are useful.
• Travel insurance – medevacs and repatriations are rarely straightforward so clarify exactly what you and the team will be covered for. For example, you may not be covered for treatment in the country of your choice.
• Risk assessment – create a risk assessment, considering the worst possible consequences from any event and its likelihood. Research local hazards. Most companies will have already created a risk matrix. Read it and feed back.
• Local hospitals/clinics – make contact if possible and research their capabilities.
• Evacuation – the insurance company will liaise with a repatriation or air ambulance company. Find out which one they will be using. Plan your evacuation route for each part of the trip with your expedition leader.
• Political – many remote areas are politically unstable. Take advice from the Foreign and Commonwealth Office very seriously. Security personnel may be recommended.

Prevention on the expedition

• Education – send an email outlining the important medical issues and hold a concise medical briefing at the start of the trip. Attention to the basics is paramount.
• Road safety – be pro-active. The highest risk of serious injury or illness is on the road. Insist on seat belts, reasonable speed, a sober driver and a serviceable vehicle. Keep medical equipment with you inside the vehicle. Swap spare keys and split up the resources between vehicles in any convoy.
• Hygiene – discuss travel basics (e.g. beware street vendors, ice cubes and hand-washed salads), handwashing, toilet site selection and disposal of waste tissue on the move.
• Water/hydration – understand your methods of supplying potable water. Encourage sensible hydration, as many will prefer to drink less to minimise urination breaks. Thirst and urine colour are good guides.

• Travellers' diarrhoea – extremely common and inconvenient if on the move. Ensure fluid balance. Often just loose stools with the change in diet. Consider early ciprofloxacin 1 g to reduce duration of symptoms. Severe vomiting, fever or blood (dysentery) will prompt evacuation. NB, other serious infections may present similarly, e.g. meningitis, malaria.
• Alcohol – most tend to abstain during the trip but the postexpedition celebration is high risk. The medic is 24 hours 'on-call' so alcohol is not advised.
• Dental – emphasise diligent hygiene. High sugar diet and fatigue lead to many problems. Warn about broken teeth on frozen snacks.
• Menstrual cycle – prepare to give advice on contraception that minimises the inconvenience of menstruation on expedition.

Specific environmental hazards

• Hypothermia – advise on disciplined layering of clothes, avoidance of sweating and high calorie intake. Early signs are apathy and poor coordination. Shivering is vital and means the patient can warm themselves. Hypothermic, non-shivering patients are seriously unwell.
• Cold injury – advise early reporting of numbness in digits, multiple types of gloves, and a buddy system to spot uncovered skin. Avoid touching metal and petrol/alcohol. Blood flow is the key so tight boots with thick socks have higher risk. Prognosis is impossible until warm water (38–42°C) immersion rewarming. Do not ever rewarm if the affected area can't be kept warm.
• Acute mountain sickness – starts for some >2500 m. Mild nausea, headaches, difficulty sleeping and lethargy are ubiquitous but most improve if allowed to acclimatise. Watch for social withdrawal and ataxia (high altitude cerebral oedema) or deterioration in exercise tolerance and fatigue (high altitude pulmonary oedema). Descent is the best treatment. Strongly consider acetazolamide (Diamox) prophylaxis.
• Animal attacks – learn about the local large predators and employ an experienced guide. Reasonable precautions may include the extra risk of a firearm (e.g. Arctic expeditions).
• Envenomation – curiosity, carelessness and poor camp-craft are normally the cause of envenomation so ask the guide to brief the team. Taking specific antivenom depends on remoteness, risk and ability to store it. Most are 'dry bites' or caused by a twig. Anaphylaxis, coagulopathy and paralysis are the risks. Read up on first aid and splintage.
• Malaria – choose the treatment carried based on local resistance and consider rapid testing kits. Emphasise how serious malaria can be and brief on prevention of bites.
• Other tropical diseases – expect lots of questions and disproportionate anxiety compared to malaria.
• Hyperthermia – confusion, ataxia, dry hot skin and muscle cramps. Obtain a temperature and immerse in water, spray with fans and/or ice packs at neck, axillae and groins. Can be very dangerous coupled with hyponatraemia from excessive hypotonic fluid intake.

36 Event medicine

Figure 36.1 Complex nature of events

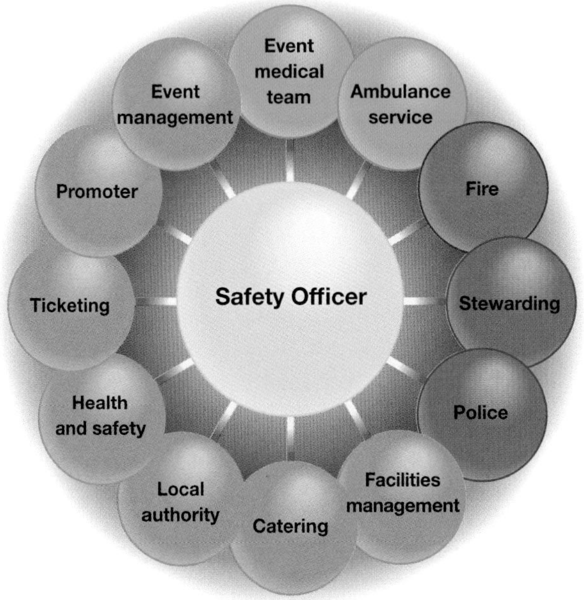

Safety Officer — Event medical team, Ambulance service, Fire, Stewarding, Police, Facilities management, Catering, Local authority, Health and safety, Ticketing, Promoter, Event management

Figure 36.2 Hierarchy of medical departments

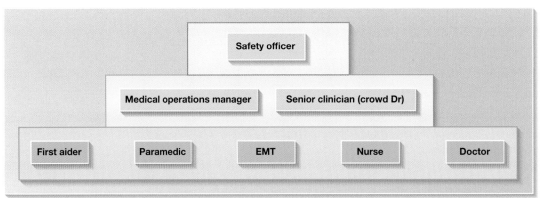

Safety officer — Medical operations manager, Senior clinician (crowd Dr) — First aider, Paramedic, EMT, Nurse, Doctor

Figure 36.3 Communication strategy

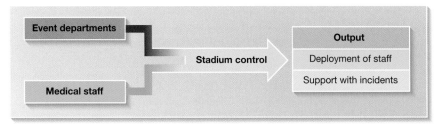

Event departments, Medical staff → Stadium control → Output: Deployment of staff, Support with incidents

Pre-hospital Emergency Medicine at a Glance, First Edition. William Seligman, Sameer Ganatra, Timothy Parker and Syed Masud.
© 2018 John Wiley & Sons, Ltd. Published 2018 by John Wiley & Sons, Ltd.

This chapter will review the organisation and management of event medicine. The principles of pre-hospital medicine apply in event medicine but it is imperative that medical staff understand the dynamic and complex nature of medical event management.

Planning

Risk assessment

All events present varying risk. The risk assessment needs to be completed for each event to identify the problems and difficulties that medical staff may face during events. This will also consider the likelihood of significant injury and the impact this will have during the event. Through the risk assessment the levels of staffing and equipment that are required can be determined. Information from previous occasions on which the event has been held is helpful in estimating the level of risk.

Staffing

The risk assessment will outline areas of difficulty and risk and lead to decisions on staffing numbers. This decision needs to be made using guidance outlined by the Sports Ground Safety Authority (SGSA) if working in sporting stadia. Relevant guidance also exists for concerts and festival sites. Staffing resources need to be adequate to maintain a safe level of cover within a venue. This will normally include a range of health professionals from doctors and paramedics to first aiders. The level of staffing and resources needs to be in keeping with the business model. All events are designed to generate revenue and therefore there may be a limit on the number of doctors that would be affordable. This needs to be considered in the assessment. Justification may be sought from senior management.

Equipment

Varying levels of equipment are required. The majority of people attending events are healthy people in search of a good day out. People will, however, get ill and require medical attention. Largely, medical care focuses around primary care and minor wounds and injuries which requires small amounts of equipment. Preparation must also be made to supply advanced life support and significant trauma care should the need arise. However, this emergency equipment should be minimal, with more focus on primary care.

Method of management

On arrival at the event, all staff need to know their role, what is expected of them and they should feel comfortable with what is requested. Demonstration of how the event will be covered throughout all areas is required. A document clearly outlining how staff will be deployed and act should a serious incident occur is essential. This allows for effective movement of staff and reassurance for senior management on how medical resources are being used. This is related to the theories presented in Chapter 7.

Training

All staff in event medicine must have relevant training. There will be a range of expertise to draw upon from the collection of staff, but this expertise must be unified. This can be achieved through regular training simulations and education sessions. Training is important to ensure staff are well rehearsed and knowledgeable about challenges that may be faced during an event. As new staff enter the workforce, training elements need to be revisited on a regular basis to ensure consistency. High fidelity simulation on-site is an excellent means to ensure a cohesive team. However, during debriefs care must be taken to ensure that people do not feel that their integrity is being questioned. A reasonably flat hierarchy is required between medical disciplines to reduce the likelihood of error.

Command and control

Figure 36.2 identifies the complex nature and the involvement of numerous departments within events. This pivots around the site safety officer who has overall responsibility for event safety. A hierarchical system is required within the management system to filter information and escalate problems. This means that only serious problems or issues reach senior management. A low level of authority is required between medical disciplines to reduce the likelihood of error.

Communication

Figure 36.1 identifies the management of communication. When dealing with highly complex events, a centre for communication is necessary. This is often identified as event control. The medical staff should be located within event control. This is to allow them to have access to other departments within the same room and will enhance and speed up communication. Any calls from security or stewarding staff will be made to the security area of event control. This can efficiently be passed to medical control for despatch of relevant medical resources. Effective methods of communication used during events are: radios (normally safe digital networks); telephone; email; face to face communication; log sheets; CCTV.

Business continuity

All events have a business purpose, even a local school fete aimed at raising money for the school. Large-scale events are held to generate revenue. Therefore, all decisions concerning medical care must consider the business, in terms of cost or reputation. A business with a good reputation will attract more business and increase profit whereas a business with a poor reputation will lose money. Excellence in customer service is paramount when working at an event. This does not mean deviation from good medical care, but in the event environment the patient becomes a customer.

Debrief and review

Throughout the course of any event, there will be a great deal of activity. It is important that appropriate debriefs occur either in written or verbal format depending on the level required. Separate debriefs may also be necessary following critical incidents. It is important to remember that as well as medical debriefs, whole event team debriefs are required. This allows feedback from medical management to senior level staff to help improve and develop the event environment and ultimately improve the customer or event owner experience.

37 Military pre-hospital emergency care

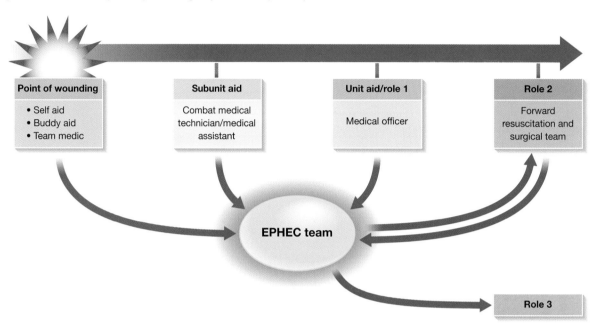

Figure 37.1 Enhanced pre-hospital emergency care team (EPHEC)

Point of wounding
- Self aid
- Buddy aid
- Team medic

Subunit aid
Combat medical technician/medical assistant

Unit aid/role 1
Medical officer

Role 2
Forward resuscitation and surgical team

EPHEC team

Role 3

Equipment: medical
- Tourniquets, FFDS, Celox
- Advanced airway equipment and ventilator
- Basic airway equipment
- Suction
- Oxygen
- IO and IV access equipment
- Fluids: blood products and crystalloid
- Multi function monitoring: HR, BP, SpO_2 and CO_2
- Defibrillator
- Thoracostomy/thoracotomy sets
- Chest seals
- Splints: cervical, pelvic and long bone
- Warming blankets and fluid warmers

Equipment: medications
- RSI drugs: induction agents, paralytics and maintenance
- Analgesia
- Tranexamic acid and calcium gluconate/chloride
- ALS drugs
- Medical emergency drugs: nebulisers, antibiotics, steroids, etc

Possible EPHEC team transport
AIR:
- CH-47 'Chinook'
- Merlin
- Puma
- Lynx
- Bell Griffin
- Sea King

Equipment: personal
- Combat clothing
- PPE: helmet, body armour, glasses, gloves
- Personal weapons: rifle and pistol
- Personal communication device/radio
- Survival equipment
- 'Down' bag: >24 hours rations, water, warm clothing, etc

Land
- Battlefield ambulance: armoured and non armoured

Sea
- LCVP (landing craft vehicle personnel)
- LCAC (landing craft air cushioned)
- Raiding craft

The EPHEC team size will also have to vary depending on the situation and resources available (e.g. doctor, nurse, 2x paramedics or doctor and paramedic)

With this range of transport resources EPHEC teams will have to be able to work in a variety of ways. 'Treating and transporting' or 'treating then transporting' and potentially switching between strategies over the course of the casualties' evacuation.

Pre-hospital Emergency Medicine at a Glance, First Edition. William Seligman, Sameer Ganatra, Timothy Parker and Syed Masud.
© 2018 John Wiley & Sons, Ltd. Published 2018 by John Wiley & Sons, Ltd.

Like its NHS counterpart, military pre-hospital emergency care is evolving. It is becoming more regulated and an increasing number of individuals have formal training in the field. The three services in the UK military have contributed individually to the speciality and have different requirements. However, the general approach for military pre-hospital care is similar, regardless of service or situation.

Process and capability

Treatment and evacuation in the military is based on the C-ABCDE paradigm and a 1-2-4 hour timeline. Ideally, this means 1 hour to reach primary surgery. If this is not possible then it is 1 hour to reach a Battlefield Advance Trauma Life Support (BATLS) qualified individual, 2 hours to reach Damage Control Surgery (DCS) and 4 hours to reach primary surgery.

The individual and team medical training that soldiers, sailors and airmen undergo facilitate the pre-hospital medical care that the military provides:

1 *Individual Aid*: each serviceman or women is trained to treat their own injuries if the situation required.
2 *Buddy–Buddy Aid*: is the process by which immediate colleagues provide medical aid.
3 *Team Medic*: is a regular soldier, sailor or airman with increased training and equipment.
4 *Combat Medical Technician or equivalent*: may be trained up-to paramedic standard and have further equipment resources.

Role 1: care at this level is usually undertaken under the guidance of a Medical Officer with at least BATLS training. This is a capability that allows field resuscitation and stabilisation and is usually integrated into the footprint of a larger unit (field force or ship).

Enhanced pre-hospital emergency care (EPHEC) teams: these are clinician-led teams of variable size and professional mix but always include a physician with advanced airway and resuscitation skills (predominantly but not universally Emergency Medicine and Anaesthetic Consultants who undertake pre-hospital care on a regular basis) and will ideally be able to provide haemostatic fluid resuscitation with the provision of blood products.

The first 'hospital' level care facility in the military medical evacuation chain is the *Role 2* which can provide DCS, has basic laboratory and imaging facilities and usually the provision of an intensive care unit holding capability. With the possibility of increased timelines, especially on entry-level operations, the military pre-hospital specialist needs additional training in the prolonged care of severely injured individuals in austere and hostile environments.

Methods of evacuation

As in the civilian sector, evacuation can be via land or air, but may include by sea. The platforms available may be tailored specifically for the evacuation purpose or have been diverted from other tasks. This necessitates the military pre-hospital specialist to be familiar with a wide range of platforms and have the flexibility to potentially swap between them during the evacuation phase. Utilisation of EPHEC teams may allow casualties to leap-frog over stages of the standard evacuation chain.

Most civilian services treat and then transfer. The ideal platform is one that allows for both treatment and transfer to occur simultaneously therefore decreasing the pre-hospital time. At present the gold standard for this is the Medical Emergency Response Team (MERT) in Afghanistan where an EPHEC team is placed on a CH-47 'Chinook', allowing 360° access and care to the patient while moving rapidly towards more advanced medical facilities.

Environment

The pre-hospital environment has both natural and man-made challenges and these are compounded in the military environment by the tactical and strategic situation. Operating in the cold and dark is difficult enough but when white light is not permitted and noise must be minimised then specialist training is required.

The non-permissive and semi-permissive environments are the most restrictive for the pre-hospital care practitioner. 'Care under fire' and 'tactical field care' are terms used in these environments for the level of care that can be provided; this may mean that just the basics are possible to maintain life prior to evacuation. Evacuation to an environment where greater care can be undertaken has to be tempered against the safety of the move. Further enemy action, improvised explosive devices or mines may lead to additional casualties which will both reduce the speed of evacuation, decrease the level of care provided to any one casualty and further 'clog' the medical chain and resources.

Future

Military pre-hospital care is developing quickly. Training requirements are similar to civilian counterparts but by necessity are broader and cross the boundaries of single service domains. As further advances are made in equipment, fluids and medications then the care of injured servicemen will improve. As non-blood oxygen carrying fluids, long-lasting clotting products and medications that have long-term stability in a wider range of temperatures are developed, then the reliance on a 'cold chain' will decrease and the scope of military pre-hospital care will broaden further.

In an ever-changing world there is the potential for military pre-hospital specialists to be involved in humanitarian operations. In areas not covered by non-government organisations, the skills of treatment and evacuation in extremely hostile environments, where those injured will also be malnourished and severely fatigued, are required. This will necessitate a further development of the specialty. Military pre-hospital care has set an impressive standard over the last decade, with patients who would have previously succumbed to their wounds making it to hospital and surviving. The challenge must continue to be met.

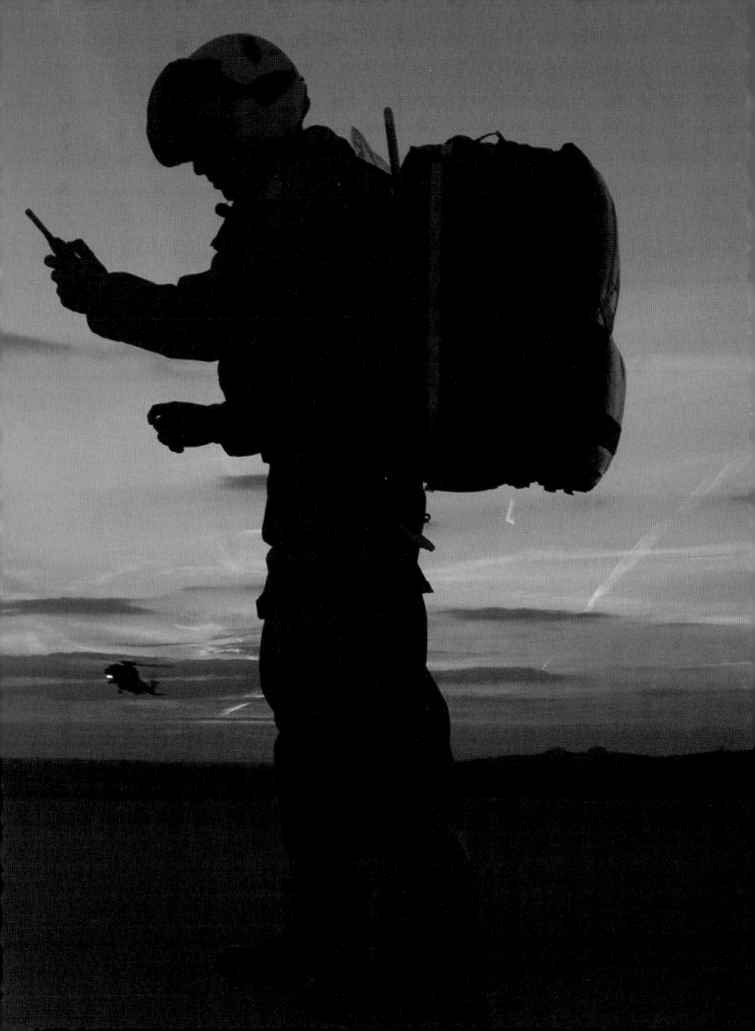

Careers in pre-hospital emergency medicine

Part 6

Chapter

38 Careers in pre-hospital emergency medicine – NHS England

Figure 38.1 Medical training pathways in PHEM

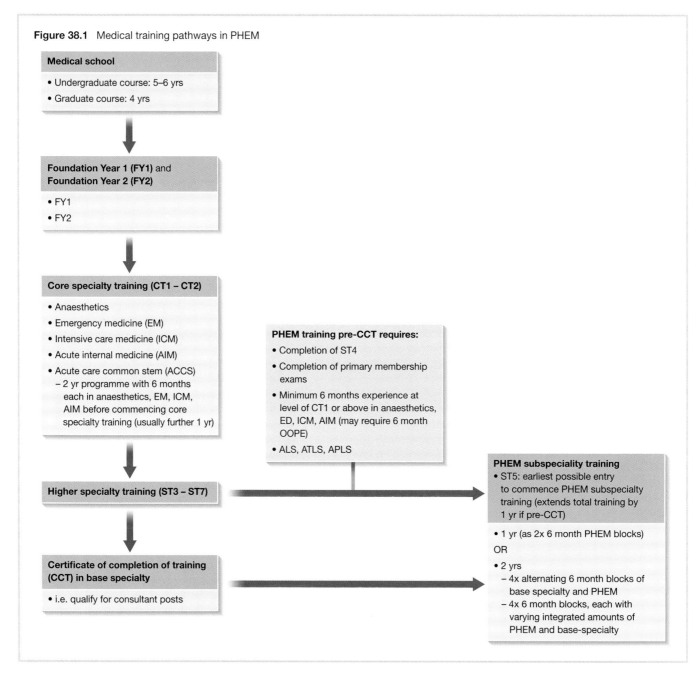

Medical school
- Undergraduate course: 5–6 yrs
- Graduate course: 4 yrs

Foundation Year 1 (FY1) and Foundation Year 2 (FY2)
- FY1
- FY2

Core specialty training (CT1 – CT2)
- Anaesthetics
- Emergency medicine (EM)
- Intensive care medicine (ICM)
- Acute internal medicine (AIM)
- Acute care common stem (ACCS)
  - 2 yr programme with 6 months each in anaesthetics, EM, ICM, AIM before commencing core specialty training (usually further 1 yr)

PHEM training pre-CCT requires:
- Completion of ST4
- Completion of primary membership exams
- Minimum 6 months experience at level of CT1 or above in anaesthetics, ED, ICM, AIM (may require 6 month OOPE)
- ALS, ATLS, APLS

Higher specialty training (ST3 – ST7)

Certificate of completion of training (CCT) in base specialty
- i.e. qualify for consultant posts

PHEM subspeciality training
- ST5: earliest possible entry to commence PHEM subspecialty training (extends total training by 1 yr if pre-CCT)

- 1 yr (as 2x 6 month PHEM blocks)
OR
- 2 yrs
  - 4x alternating 6 month blocks of base specialty and PHEM
  - 4x 6 month blocks, each with varying integrated amounts of PHEM and base-specialty

Pre-hospital Emergency Medicine at a Glance, First Edition. William Seligman, Sameer Ganatra, Timothy Parker and Syed Masud.
© 2018 John Wiley & Sons, Ltd. Published 2018 by John Wiley & Sons, Ltd.

Medical careers in pre-hospital emergency medicine

Pre-hospital emergency medicine has only recently been recognised by the General Medical Council (GMC) as a specific subspecialty in its own right and as such the following details are subject to change. Particularly of note are ongoing efforts to include an approved training pathway for General Practice trainees.

Training pathways

Pre-hospital emergency medicine was initially recognised as a subspecialty of Emergency Medicine and Anaesthesia by the GMC on 20 July 2011; subspecialty status was later granted for Intensive Care Medicine (ICM) and Acute Internal Medicine (AIM) on 1 October 2013. PHEM now has an approved curriculum and training structure with a national selection process administered by the Intercollegiate Board for Training in Pre-Hospital Emergency Medicine (IBTPHEM).

Doctors, regardless of their chosen base specialty, must have completed ST4 training and have successfully passed their primary membership examinations to be eligible for PHEM training to commence at the earliest in ST5. They must also have accrued a minimum of 6 months' experience, at the level of CT1 or above, in each of emergency medicine, anaesthetics and ICM; a lack of any of these may be compensated for by a 6 month placement taken as part of an Out-of-Programme Experience (OOPE).

Scope for practise before ST5 has become extremely limited in the UK with the introduction of the GMC's Approved Practice Settings (APS), which limits the ability of doctors to work outside their usual practice setting until they have a minimum of 5 years' post-graduate training. PHEM subspecialty training itself requires 1 year whole-time equivalent (WTE); that is, a total of a year's worth of training which may be taken in a single block, or integrated with ongoing base specialty training over 2 years.

Career structures

Workforce estimates indicate the need for around 200–250 full-time equivalent PHEM consultant posts. As each consultant will have a minimum 50% commitment to their base specialty (i.e. an emergency medicine consultant will spend at least half of their working time in the Emergency Department and their remaining working time in a PHEM capacity), this equates to the need for 600–750 PHEM consultants nationally. At the time of writing, increasing numbers of training posts are becoming available to reflect this demand.

Considerations

A career in PHEM is highly challenging; working conditions are often difficult, in uncontrolled and dangerous environments, with limited equipment and advanced care delivered regardless of the weather and time of day and isolated from additional support. Decision making is time critical and delays cost lives. Many candidates find the psychological impact of being on-scene at the site of major trauma intensely difficult to deal with, especially when involving children. There is intense scrutiny of management decisions throughout training and in ongoing practise, and patients suffering devastating injury will frequently die despite the very best efforts made. This makes a career in PHEM in equal parts challenging but intensely rewarding, and the balance lies very much with the individual. It is also imperative that doctors are content in their chosen base specialty, as a significant portion of time is spent in this role.

Paramedic careers in pre-hospital emergency medicine

The ambulance service in the UK has experienced significant pressure in recent years to meet the increasing healthcare requirements of the community. The number of 999 calls has risen nationally by one-third in the past 5 years and in a constant attempt to meet the annual increase in pre-hospital service demand the role of the paramedic has evolved. There has been an arguable shift in improving clinical performance and extending clinical skills.

Paramedic education has moved in line with other allied health professions with education now at Higher Education Institutes for existing (non-paramedic) staff and those joining the profession for the first time. The universities work closely with ambulance trusts to provide courses leading to Health and Care Professions Council registration as paramedics. The increasing numbers of paramedics with higher education qualifications is creating a workforce with enhanced clinical skills and autonomy, reflecting the diversity of ambulance service work.

Careers within the ambulance service for qualified paramedics focus on subspecialties of pre-hospital care. These new advanced practitioner roles range from specialties in primary care (a reflection for the need to deliver healthcare to the patient) to critical care roles (delivering advanced life support beyond the scope of a paramedic). Nationally, variation still exists in these practitioner roles, as does the ever-changing environment for paramedics.

Degree-educated paramedics are increasingly creating roles within other healthcare settings, working alongside other allied healthcare professionals in equivalent roles. This area of practice is currently being seen in regional deaneries where pre-hospital specialist paramedics are being recruited to Doctorate in Clinical Practice (DClinP) courses, developing the practitioner to lead innovative and effective evidence-based healthcare.

References

Chapter 1
Andersen D. *The history of prehospital and retrieval medicine.* Lecture at Social Media and Critical Care Conference, 2013.

Chapter 3
http://www.ncepod.org.uk/2007report2/Downloads/SIP_summary.pdf

http://www.nhshistory.net/darzilondon.pdf

https://www.gov.uk/government/uploads/system/uploads/attachment_data/file/228836/7432.pdf

https://www.nao.org.uk/wp-content/uploads/2010/02/0910213.pdf

Chapter 4
Bell A. *et al.* Physician Response Unit – a feasibility study of an initiative to enhance the delivery of pre-hospital emergency medical care. *Resuscitation* 2006;69:389–93.

http://content.digital.nhs.uk/catalogue/PUB11062/ambu-serv-eng-2012-2013-rep.pdf

https://www.england.nhs.uk/wp-content/uploads/2014/10/5yfv-web.pdf

www.nhs.uk/NHSEngland/keogh-review/Pages/urgent-and-emergency-care-review.aspx

Chapter 6
Nutbeam T, Boylan M. *ABC of Prehospital Emergency Medicine.* Wiley Blackwell, 2013.

Chapter 14
Apfelbaum J, Hagberg C, Caplan R, Blitt C, Connis R, Nickinovich D. et al. Practice Guidelines for Management of the Difficult Airway. *Anesthesiology* 2013;118(2):251–270.

Berry J. A Tight Squeeze. *EMS Airway Clinic.* Nov 2011.

Chrimes N. The Vortex: a universal 'high-acuity implementation tool' for emergency airway management. *British Journal of Anaesthesia* 2016;117(suppl 1):i20–i27.

Frerk C. et al. Difficult Airway Society 2015 Guidelines For Management Of Unanticipated Difficult Intubation In Adults. *British Journal of Anaesthesia* 115.6, 2015;827–848.

Walls R, Murphy M. *Manual of emergency airway management.* 4th ed. Philadelphia: Wolters Kluwer/Lippincott Williams & Wilkins Heath; 2012.

https://academic.oup.com/bja/article/115/6/827/241440/Difficult-Airway-Society-2015-guidelines-for

https://www.das.uk.com/files/das2015intubation_guidelines.pdf

Chapter 16
Hirshberg A, *et al.* Minimizing dilutional coagulopathy in exsanguinating hemorrhage: a computer simulation. *J Trauma* 2003;54:454–63.

Sander GE, Giles TD. Ximelagatran: Light at the End of the Tunnel or the Next Tunnel? *Am J Geriatr Cardiol.* 2004;13(4).

Chapter 18
Lockey D, Crewdson K, Davies G. Traumatic cardiac arrest: who are the survivors? *Ann Emerg Med* 2006;48:240–4.

Chapter 24
http://www.frca.co.uk/Documents/172%20Trauma%20in%20pregnancy.pdf

Paterson-Brown S, Howell C (Eds) *Managing Obstetric Emergencies and Trauma: The MOET Course Manual.* 3rd Edition. Cambridge: Cambridge University Press, 2016.

Chapter 25
Griffiths R, Mehta M. Frailty and anaesthesia: what we need to know. *BJA Education* 2014; 14:273–77.

Spoors C, Kiff K (Eds) *Training in Anaesthesia (Oxford Specialty Training).* Oxford: Oxford University Press, 2010.

www.acep.org/Content.aspx?id=7974

www.sign.ac.uk/pdf/sign111.pdf

Chapter 32
Moss R, *et al.* Minimal patient handling: a faculty of prehospital care consensus statement. *Emerg Med J* 2013;30:1065–6.

Sources

Chapter 8
Figure 8.1 Thames Valley Air Ambulance.

Figure 8.2 Andrew Linnett/MOD.

https://commons.wikimedia.org/wiki/File%3ARAF_Chinook_Mark_6_Helicopter_MOD_45158783.jpg

Used under the Open Government Licence v1.0 (OGL).

https://www.nationalarchives.gov.uk/doc/open-government-licence/version/1/;

Figure 8.3 Holbery N, Newcombe P. Emergency Nursing at a Glance (2016). Reproduced with permission of John Wiley & Sons;

Figure 8.4 Curimedia | P H O T O G R A P H Y

https://commons.wikimedia.org/wiki/File%3ABeechcraft_C90GTx_King_Air_Hawker_Beechcraft_N2060K_(9334610247).jpg

Used under CC BY 2.0 (http://creativecommons.org/licenses/by/2.0)], via Wikimedia Commons;

Figure 8.5 Andrew Thomas, Shrewsbury, UK

https://commons.wikimedia.org/w/index.php?curid=37522057 Used under CC BY-SA 2.0 https://creativecommons.org/licenses/by-sa/2.0/

Pre-hospital Emergency Medicine at a Glance, First Edition. William Seligman, Sameer Ganatra, Timothy Parker and Syed Masud.
© 2018 John Wiley & Sons, Ltd. Published 2018 by John Wiley & Sons, Ltd.

Chapter 15

Figure 15.1 Airway obstruction: Leach RM. *Critical Care Medicine at a Glance* (2014). Reproduced with permission of John Wiley & Sons.

Tension pneumothorax: Massive haemothorax; Open pneumothorax; Flail chest: Hughes T, Cruickshank J. *Adult Emergency Medicine at a Glance* (2011). Reproduced with permission of John Wiley & Sons.

Cardiac tamponade: Holbery N, Newcombe P. *Emergency Nursing at a Glance* (2016). Reproduced with permission of John Wiley & Sons.

Chapter 20

Figure 20.2 Diffuse axonal injury: By SBarnes – Karen Tong, CC BY-SA 3.0, https://commons.wikimedia.org/w/index.php?curid=5874994.

Intraparenchymal haemorrhage: By MD Computed Tomography diagnostic Team (WWW) [Copyrighted free use], via Wikimedia Commons.

Epidural hematoma: By Jpogi – Own work, CC BY-SA 3.0, https://commons.wikimedia.org/w/index.php?curid=20339304.

Subdural haematoma: By James Heilman, MD – Own work, CC BY-SA 3.0, https://commons.wikimedia.org/w/index.php?curid=19364350.

Index

Pre-hospital Emergency Medicine at a Glance, First Edition. William Seligman, Sameer Ganatra, Timothy Parker and Syed Masud.
© 2018 John Wiley & Sons, Ltd. Published 2018 by John Wiley & Sons, Ltd.